THE
ART OF
GENERAL
PRACTICE

SOFT SKILLS
TO SURVIVE AND THRIVE

D1438573

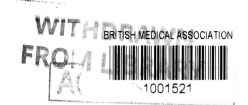

For Rosie

THE

SOFT SKILLS

ART OF

TO SURVIVE

GENERAL

AND THRIVE

PRACTICE

DAVID BARTLETT
Formerly a GP in Olney, Bucks

Scion

© Scion Publishing Limited, 2018

ISBN 9781911510192

First published 2018

A CIP catalogue record for this book is available from the British Library.

Scion Publishing Limited

The Old Hayloft, Vantage Business Park, Bloxham Road, Banbury OX16 9UX, UK

www.scionpublishing.com

Important Note from the Publisher

The information contained within this book was obtained by Scion Publishing Ltd from sources believed by us to be reliable. However, while every effort has been made to ensure its accuracy, no responsibility for loss or injury whatsoever occasioned to any person acting or refraining from action as a result of information contained herein can be accepted by the authors or publishers.

Although every effort has been made to ensure that all owners of copyright material have been acknowledged in this publication, we would be pleased to acknowledge in subsequent reprints or editions any omissions brought to our attention.

Registered names, trademarks, etc. used in this book, even when not marked as such, are not to be considered unprotected by law.

Use the free Learning Diary app from FourteenFish to record your notes and reflection as you read this book.

www.fourteenfish.com/app

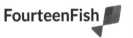

Typeset by Medlar Publishing Solutions Pvt Ltd, India

Printed in the UK by Ashford Colour Press

Last digit is the print number: 10 9 8 7 6 5 4 3 2 1

Contents

SECTION II

Looking after number one, *or* Stayin' alive

Preface

I've loved my career in general practice. It has been full of interest, although there have naturally been times of sadness, stress and fatigue. But overall it has been a real privilege. So many people have chosen to put their trust in me, to share with me their painful emotions and life stories, and many have become friends. Not of course in the close sense, but there has been a mutual interest in each other's lives and families which has made some consultations feel little like work.

In this book, I have tried to say what I think can make a successful career in general practice more likely. It will first require attention to your own health and wellbeing. I have said to many patients that I owe a responsibility to myself so that I can be in the best possible state to be of help to them. There are many self-help books on resilience and plenty of literature in the various training materials for GPs in training. I'm not trying to add to, nor summarise, what others may have said. I just offer a few key ideas that I believe have made a difference to me throughout my career.

General practice is not primarily about the wellbeing of the doctor, but how to provide the best possible care for the patient. If some of what I say seems idealistic I can only say that if you don't aim high, you will inevitably settle for the mediocre. This will have various negative effects. You will enjoy your career less, your patients will feel less well cared for and are more likely to complain about you. If such complaints come often and are about more serious matters, the stress you will experience will be enormous. I believe that working hard to practise the art of medicine is good for patients but self-preserving as well.

I haven't attempted to be comprehensive in this short book. I have wanted to stimulate thought and provide something to interact with, as you consider your own practice of medicine. We are all different and I recognise that I have a particular personality type and life experience. However, all of us can change, adapt and grow and I hope these pages will facilitate your own development.

The first section of the book is on what one might loosely call the craft of general practice. It doesn't contain up-to-date guidelines on the diagnosis and management of medical conditions, since there are plenty of other resources for that. I did, however, want to stress the soft skills of general practice, which are so necessary. In many ways they are an outworking of thoughtfulness and empathy, but which add greatly to one's enjoyment and skill in the practice of medicine.

The second section has additional material which I hope will help you build resilience. Since general practice is a demanding career with constant changes from above, changes in guidelines and the changeableness of patients, we need strong foundations to survive. And we also need the ability to recognise when things are getting out of control, and to adapt as necessary. I hope some of these ideas prove of value to you.

Many colleagues have inspired and helped me. But also, I have been greatly helped by reading articles and books and throughout this book you will see many references to some of them. I must add my apologies where I have forgotten the origin of my thinking, gleaned from so many sources through my career.

I wish you well in what must be one of the best jobs in the world.

David Bartlett
February 2018

Acknowledgements

I owe a debt of thanks to so many people for knowingly or, more likely, incidentally, affecting me and the way I practise medicine. As I age I realise more and more how much I owe to my mother and her ability to relate so well to all manner of people with kindness and thoughtfulness.

My trainer Bernard Baillon was a calming influence early on in my career and I have been blessed with several partners at Cobbs Garden Surgery. I'm grateful most notably to my former senior partner, Nigel Swallow, who conducted my interview for partnership in his back garden whilst sharing his home-brew beer with me. He was always polite, straightforward and had an impish sense of humour. I'm also grateful to Brian Partridge who was my partner for 30 years and whose enthusiasm for general practice is undimmed.

Like all GPs I have learned so much from the hundreds of patients I have had the privilege of caring for, and I'm grateful that many of them have become friends. I would also like to thank my secretary Jane Folds for reading all my outpourings and who was generous in her comments.

Lastly, I'm thankful for my family who have been with me and supported me throughout my GP career. For my wife Biddy (aka Liz), who has worked alongside me as a practice nurse, and who still receives far more presents from patients than I ever received. And for our daughters Sarah and Hannah who are our best friends and despite being in their thirties, still want to join us on holidays.

SECTION I

Soft skills

We are drowning in a plethora of guidelines, formularies, data collection and QOF. Add to that the growth of computer-based diagnostic programs and referral guidelines, and it feels as though the practice of medicine is becoming a kind of 'paint by numbers'. It seems there's little room for what one might call the 'impressionism' of doctoring, and for the type of practice that needs humanity and emotional intelligence.

The chapters in this first section aim to place the doctor–patient relationship at the centre. They attempt to foster the use of simple soft skills in our daily practice. If done well, I believe that everyone wins – the patient, the NHS and the doctor.

1

Greeting the patient

None of us can avoid first impressions. Although at times they may completely mislead us, with growing experience they can become very valuable.

How do you call patients into your consulting room? Over the years there have been many systems, from bells and buzzers, to names appearing on a screen, to receptionists calling, or even the outgoing patient simply saying, "Next" as they walk past the waiting room (as was the case in my early years in practice). I'd like to make a case for going to the waiting room yourself and calling the patient. I believe there are many benefits which outweigh the objections.

The moment you call the patient and see them, you are beginning your assessment. You can look at their body language as they rise from their seat and subsequently sit down in your consulting room. You can see whether they are accompanied or alone. Some patients begin 'talking' to you as they enter, perhaps groaning a little or huffing or looking to be genuinely out of breath. And then there is the all-important gait – Parkinsonian, antalgic, hobbling; so much information can be gathered before the patient enters your room.

Remember that the patient is sizing you up too. Noting your appearance and attitude, and perhaps deciding whether or not they can tell you that embarrassing something that is bugging them, or whether you are sending signals of being stressed or too busy.

Then there is the greeting. What, if anything, do you say as they enter? Of course, much will depend upon how well, if at all, you know one another, but it's a human skill to be able to adapt to people and, as a GP, you should aim to be a 'people person'. So what of the GP who gets as far as calling the patient but then charges off to their room, leaving the patient trailing in their wake? Having sat in waiting rooms myself, that just looks and feels rude. If someone opened the front door to you and simply walked into the heart of the house leaving you to follow, you would think it odd. Having greeted the patient you may well walk ahead of them, but why not stand aside and allow them to go in the room first? My mum would say it's basic manners. Maybe a neurosurgeon can get away with gruffness (although that's hardly a virtue), but that's not for us.

But what to say? I employ various greetings, from the casual "Come along" or "Good to see you" (if you mean it!) to, "Ah the dynamic duo... you've come with your bodyguard I see". Of course, all such attempts at levity may fall dreadfully flat if it's just not your style, but at least find a vocabulary that begins to convey that you don't regard the patient as a nuisance. You don't need to start the consultation on the way in but at least talk, be friendly, greet children appropriately: "Hiya sweetie" might make the examination of his painful ear in three minutes' time somewhat easier.

I imagine your first response to this will be along the lines of: 'But I don't have time, I can write up the notes while the patient is coming from the waiting room'. True, but is that so important? If it has been a particularly long and complicated consultation I favour the option of dictating the consultation for the secretary to write up. Even the longest mental health consultation in general practice can be dictated within a small number of minutes. And 'saving time' is a relative concept. It's rather like overtaking that slow driver in front of you; by the end of the journey you may have 'saved' two minutes, but at what risk or cost? In our daily practice, I don't think waiting in the consulting room relentlessly looking at my computer screen is the best use of my time, plus it is dull and claustrophobic. So many patients have complained to me of their doctor gazing at the screen as they walk in, making them feel as though they are intruding. It's not a great way to begin a consultation. So why not stretch your legs, since every bit of exercise helps. Wear a pedometer to see what difference it really makes.

Do yourself (and your patient) a favour. Go get 'em.

───────────── **For reflection** ─────────────

- To what extent do you feel the way you greet a patient contributes to the doctor–patient relationship?

- What impression do you think the patient forms of you as they enter from the waiting room?

- Do you change your greeting to the patient when you are running late?

2

More greetings

Greeting the doctor

A colleague of mine in his first practice was somewhat unnerved by the greeting he received from the patient as he entered the consulting room, "Hello young man". The young doctor had not been in the practice many months and felt rather belittled and inadequate as the smooth-talking businessman sat down and waited for my colleague's opening question.

There are many situations that can unnerve us. This is especially so in our early years in practice when many of our patients are older, frequently wiser and simply more experienced then we are at doing life. How should we respond? Naturally there is no one right way, but it is important that we develop ways which will ultimately lead to rapport and connection with the patient, and enable them to trust and value our judgement.

So, you have received the greeting, "Hello young man", or "… young lady". How would you respond? Some ideas:

- The clever dick approach – "That's very kind of you, and how are you old fella?"

- The uber-professional – "How can I help you?", thereby ignoring the greeting

- The get-off-to-a-bad-start approach – "I'm not as young as I look, which sadly cannot be said for you"

- The friendly approach – "It's a while since I've been called that".

What did the patient mean by the greeting, if indeed there was any conscious or sub-conscious meaning? Was he trying to establish a priority in the relationship, with the patient running the show and the young doctor merely a pawn or gateway into further medical help? Was the patient arrogant and self-confident or perhaps even somewhat embarrassed by having to confide in such a young person? Does he greet all young people this way by the nature of his work as a lecturer, teacher or trainer of some kind, and merely 'forgot' himself? There's seldom one explanation to anything that is said like this!

In general practice these situations happen in a moment, and one relies upon reflexes and instinct. The sort of reflection engaged in above takes a little more time, but it repays the effort. Everything matters in a consultation. Gradually over time you should aim to develop a style which maximises the benefits of patients consulting you and enhances your own enjoyment and satisfaction in a job well done. It is well worth the effort.

Couple therapy

Many GPs find it a little unsettling when patients attend with their partner, family member or friend. However, often there is significance to it. How best to greet them? I confess I attempt a little levity with most of my patients, since I generally know them well and I've been around a long time. My favourites are:

- "Ah it's Bonnie and Clyde"

- "And how are the happy couple?"

- "May I say welcome to the dynamic duo"

- "Ah, I see you've brought your bodyguard"

- "You realise that you'll be charged double on the way out?"

All such comments are of course to be avoided if you do not know the couple or sense that the humour gene is lacking (in my experience that will apply to fairly few patients, although perhaps that is one of the groups of patients who avoid me). And if *your* humour gene is lacking, definitely don't try it, but then how do you survive in medicine without some humour?

Greetings to be super-cautious with are:

- "Ah, it's Little and Large"

- "Ah, two fat ladies"

- "Uh-oh, this looks ominous"

- "Not you two again!"

But there is another side to this; *why* have they come together?

- They may be expecting worrying news and want to be present together to hear it.

- The non-patient partner wants to make sure the patient tells the truth, the whole truth and nothing but the truth.

- The non-patient partner wears the trousers.

- The patient may be hard of hearing.

- The non-patient may be super-caring and devoted.

- They may want to gang up on you.

- They may want to sneak an extra opinion from you, on the non-patient.

- You may have asked them to attend together…. and forgotten!

- They may do everything together anyway.

Generally you should make the most of the situation. I recall a particular female patient who was a great trial to me and who usually presented in each consultation with several different problems. Now, patients arriving in twos can be a challenge, but I was always relieved when she attended with her husband. Although sometimes the husband took the supportive stance of trying to make me take the situation more seriously than I appeared to, more often than not after some minutes beyond the allotted ten, he would give his wife the "come on, the doctor hasn't got all day", which I confess I was thinking but didn't feel it would be very helpful to say.

It can also be very useful to use the supporter to confirm details of what the patient has said, and what you have said to the patient. Don't assume, however, that the patient is giving you carte blanche to break confidentiality. Thus, throughout the consultation you may want to check with the patient that they are happy for such and such a subject to be discussed. This is particularly pertinent in that difficult mid-teen age group when discussing lifestyle issues. Many a parent who boldly states that I may ask their offspring anything because "they tell me everything", would be surprised to hear that in a subsequent consultation their child brought a school friend with them and not the parent, because they didn't want mum to know.

And more and more. All to say that there is an awful lot going on in GP consultations which is why they are so endlessly fascinating.

─────────────── **For reflection** ───────────────

- Are there particular types and ages of patients that you struggle with? What might you do differently? How might you adapt?

- Have you had any difficulty with couples who attend together?

- Are there patients who intimidate you? What might you do in response?

3

Routines

Some years ago, I was with our youngest daughter in the lovely small coastal village of Cavtat. It lies just a few miles south of Dubrovnik on the Dalmatian coast of Croatia. We decided to hire two deck-chairs on the promenade overlooking the spectacular small cruise ships anchored nearby. No sooner had we paid for them and set them up when the young man who had taken our money and given us the receipt came over to us. "Tickets please", he said in a rather serious heavily accented voice. My daughter and I looked at each other and smiled, assuming he was having a joke, but no, he wanted to check that we had paid for the deckchairs. When I light-heartedly reminded him that we had bought the tickets from him less than two minutes previously, he rather frostily replied, "Just routine", in the same guttural, deadpan way. We often reminisce about the event and frequently impersonate the "just routine" when something rather obvious has just been said.

Routines are such a valuable part of daily life and without them chaos would reign. From cleaning our teeth, to driving a car, to the daily practice of medicine, routines determine much of our behaviour. But in our consultations, they can work against us.

The routine baby check

I generally enjoy the baby six-week check, and especially when the babe is the first child. Often both parents attend, and although it can take forever for those poppers to be gently opened by the tentative parent, I often feel in a relaxed mood and seldom are there major problems.

On one memorable occasion, I proceeded with my spiel and routine examination, starting by holding the baby's hands and carefully lifting little Oscar to confirm the Moro reflex. And so the examination proceeded until the triumphant conclusion and proclamation by me that Oscar was perfect in every way. But then a quizzical look greeted me from mum, "But is he meant to have six fingers and six toes on both sides?" I was momentarily flustered before rather feebly blurting out something along the lines of that being an above average situation!

Autopilot

Although routines both in history taking and examination are important, we must guard against the potential problem of being in, what can appear to the patient at least, autopilot mode. This is especially a danger with the overuse of templates on the computer. We can rattle off questions about diet and smoking, alcohol intake and family history, whilst all the time interacting with the computer far more than engaging with the patient. Similarly, we can be so focused upon getting to the end of the consultation that we may miss cues that the patient has offered us. Perhaps it's analogous to the strange situation of when we have been driving on a familiar route and yet can recall virtually nothing of the journey.

Not only might we miss important clinical matters but I suspect the patient can tell when we are in autopilot mode. Clues that we are in that mode would be impatient attempts to butt in to the patient's conversation, or asking questions that bear little relation to what the patient has just said, or worse, asking a question which the patient has already answered. You will have heard radio or television interviews where the interviewer hasn't listened to the interviewee's response; does that ever happen in your consultations? Tapping away and looking at the computer is so common now that sadly many patients have come to expect it. They might as well have consulted Google, or asked Alexa or Siri.

Take histories like a spinner

"Do you suffer with headaches? Which side are they on? What do they feel like? Do you feel sick with them? Is your vision affected?" And so on… We can be so keen to get our standard questions out that the patient can feel exhausted and indeed might even shut down, to the extent that they cannot recall what they would normally be able to tell us, were they given breathing space.

In cricketing terms, we should probably aim to be spinners who vary their pace and approach, rather than fiery fast bowlers. And also, remember that cricketers have a mini break after six balls have been bowled. The good bowler observes the way the batsman is playing before deciding upon how the next ball should be delivered. If you are too stuck in a routine, you may miss the unusual answer that you have just been given, and which may require a different line of questioning. The consultation is an unscripted live event, and needs a living, breathing, responsive doctor to make the most of it.

"It's only a cough"

The 3-month-old had been added to the end of my list. It was yet another coughing baby. 'Just routine'. My spiel was all ready to be delivered before I'd even examined him, "It's a virus….". I opened the door and invited them in. Towering above the little chap in his buggy I briefly noted that he looked half asleep and was neither breathless, wheezy nor coughing. Nonetheless I went through the usual examination and almost casually said to mum that he seemed to have been half asleep the whole time he was in the consultation. "Oh, he always looks like that." Half asleep? Eyes not fully closed and not ever fully open? It was slow to dawn on me, but at least it eventually did. He had congenital ptosis, a condition I had never seen, but which in retrospect was easy to spot. Of course, I looked it up that day and referred him promptly, since delayed referral can result in significantly impaired sight.

I reflected upon all the mothers I had spoken to over the years who had rung me about their baby and their cough. I had often given advice over the phone and not seen them. If ever there was a situation which confirmed to me the caution I feel we should have over the development of more and more triage systems done over the phone, it was this one consultation. It seems to me that not even a cough should be 'just routine'. It is a classic reminder of one of the challenges of general practice; staying alert to the sheer variety of causes, conditions and situations that face us that can get lost in routine practice. And it is perhaps one of the key things that distinguishes primary care from that of hospital practice.

────────────── **For reflection** ──────────────

- When might routines be most useful in medical practice?

- Think about your consulting posture. If you have a tendency to look at the computer more than the patient, what practical steps might you take to reach some kind of balance?

- Do you need to slow down (or perhaps even speed up) in your history taking?

- Think of clinical situations when autopilot mode might be potentially unhelpful.

- What is your approach to telephone consultations?

4

One consultation, one problem

There are certain phrases that irritate me, and this is one of them. I know why some practices display this sign prominently in the waiting room, along with the latest figures of non-attendees for appointments. It is perceived as a way to manage demand and in turn to cope with the stress of practice. But is it the best way? And does such signposting facilitate doctor–patient relationships, and create a combined 'we're in this together' approach for the practice population and its staff? Now of course we must manage demand, but I believe there are unintended consequences of such an assertive and adversarial approach.

But what is to be done with the patient who comes in with the proverbial list? It is only in Whitehall that there is the perception that the average patient who wants to see a GP simply has one very specific problem that needs addressing, and can be dealt with in one simple way. A horrible sore throat? Easy, either give antibiotics or advice. Next patient please! But any practising GP knows that no surgery is like that. Our work is considerably more complex, nuanced and varied.

The reality is that human beings are remarkable biological systems, with millions of chemical reactions going on within them at any one time. However, we are also social, emotional, spiritual and physical beings. Our complementary and alternative 'colleagues' may have little evidence base to support their practice but they at least do think in holistic terms, even if the conclusions they come to and the advice they give are not what we might support.

One of the challenges and fascinations of the GP consultation is knowing how far to take each aspect of a patient's presenting (or even hidden) problems, *at that particular consultation*. And then how many of the listed problems inter-relate.

OK, we've prevaricated enough. Mrs Jones has a list. Help!

In approaching the patient with multiple issues, much will depend upon how well you know the patient, especially in terms of negotiating how many issues to attempt to help with, and recognising that some may have a very quick answer. Here are a few ideas that may help you deal with Mrs Jones and her list.

- If the patient starts by telling you that they have a few matters to discuss, you have an advantage. At that point ask for a quick rundown of them so that *together* you can make a judgement on what can realistically be addressed on this occasion. "What would you most like help with today? Let's focus on that and see how we get on."

- If, however, after spending ten minutes on what you thought was the sole problem, the patient unexpectedly goes on to say that there are a couple of other problems to discuss… don't sigh! Politely and warmly advise them that you would like to help, but that alas you have run out of time. However, ask them briefly to say what they are. Make a quick judgement as to whether it is important clinically to try to manage any of the problems now, or more likely, that you would like to give more proper attention to them next time.

- Make a judgement as to whether any of the additional problems need a consultation soon, and decide whether to squeeze the patient in, whilst gently advising them that if you have squeezed them in, you won't be able to spend long at that next consultation, if that is indeed the case.

- It is perfectly acceptable in general practice to *partially* deal with problems during any one consultation, and not necessarily in the traditional order (e.g. history, examination then special investigations). Perhaps suggest a blood test that you may have wanted the patient to have in light of their symptoms, or maybe for them to keep a symptom diary, or perhaps to come back to you with the sequence and more detail of their symptoms written down (if you've ever been a patient you will know how hard it is to recall your story). In other words, useful things that can buy you time and dissuade the patient from feeling that you are not interested.

- It's amazing how often problems and symptoms resolve themselves. In the days of being on call from home after evening surgery I gradually learnt to delay a too immediate response to some patients. Depending upon what symptoms were being presented and how troublesome they were, after taking the history on the phone, I would gently say that I was busy at that precise moment (having my tea, reading a bedtime story, watching the news – I didn't give the detail to the patient, obviously) but that I would ring back 30–45 minutes later. I asked if that approach was acceptable to them and virtually without exception it was. Time and again the sting had been taken out of the situation when I called back and I was able to suggest waiting until the next day, by which time in many situations the problem had completely settled. A similar approach may well be helpful with the multi-list patient, and I would suggest you try a comment such as, "Can we just see how problems 3 and 4 go over the next few days and if they are still an issue we can try to deal with them next time?' If you attempt to deal with all of the problems immediately you give yourself a real challenge. Some of them will quite likely sort themselves out unaided by you, if given sufficient time. Sometimes it's just enough that the patient knows that *you* know they have multiple problems. A touch of empathy and/or sympathy was all that was needed. And never forget the GP's best friend – *time*, that great healer.

- If blood tests have been arranged, you can reasonably say that you would need to have some kind of further contact with the patient, but that would need to be after a week or so, thus giving you more breathing space.

- It's tempting to suggest making a double appointment next time, and there will be occasions when this is appropriate, but be careful of doing that too often. You are training yourself and the patient to effectively and appropriately work within the constraints of the system that exists.

I admit that working as an occasional locum makes some elements of this approach more difficult, although depending upon the type of locum, not wholly impossible.

─────────────── **For reflection** ───────────────

- What strategies do you have for coping with multiple problems during one consultation?

- Do you feel you have to completely unpack the detail of each problem or can you find ways to partially address the matter in hand and use time as a tool?

- If you work as a locum how might you approach the patient with a list?

5

Don't say that!

There aren't many specific details I recall from my medical school teaching but I do remember one adage that has stood me in good stead. 'Never say never' and 'never say always'. Often this was taught in the context of a patient asking about their treatment and the likelihood of success or failure.

Just this afternoon I saw a patient who had been to see a private cosmetic doctor. He had told her emphatically that his treatment would definitely cure her melasma on the face. Whilst there may be a good chance that the treatment might work (at least temporarily), it is bold and probably misleading to say that it *always* works. And similarly, in response to a question about the possibility of improvement it is generally wise to avoid saying that such an event would *never* ever occur. Naturally there is nuance to take account of, but in general the advice I was given was wise.

It got me thinking about things that we should avoid saying to our patients. Here's my top three.

1. "There's nothing more I can do for you"

Naturally I understand what the doctor may be implying. She may be answering a question from a patient who has not responded to treatment for an as yet undiagnosed condition (in the current jargon, 'medically unexplained'). But the impression given to the patient is of a doctor with a closed mind-set, thinking only in straight lines. It could well be the case that the doctor may not be able to think of an alternative drug or procedure. But to suggest that *nothing* can be done reinforces the sense of hopelessness and helplessness that some of our patients feel.

Maybe you can't do any more clinically, but that isn't to say that the avenues of finding relief and adaptation to whatever it is the patient is contending with, are exhausted. As James McCormick puts it in his wonderful book, *The Doctor: father figure or plumber*[1] (still very relevant although published in 1979), "health is the successful adaptation to disability".

There is always help to be had in terms of adaptation. And indeed, there may be someone else who is in a better position to help, in which case the sentiment of 'nothing I can do' is literally accurate, but it is just pejorative to say so. Patients always need to be offered hope, not false hope of cure, but hope that symptoms can be to some degree relieved, and that although recovery may not come, coping is nearly always possible, although it may be hugely challenging.

We know that many of our patients would feel better if they were less self-focused, and that giving them encouragement and permission to make someone else's day may sound rather 'New Age-like', but it is fundamentally true. Many times, I have seen patients

---

1 · *The Doctor: father figure or plumber*, James McCormick, 1979, Croom Helm Ltd, Dundee

'recover' by taking up a new interest, or finding love, or starting a new job, or taking on the care of someone else. It's an example of what the old Scottish theologian Thomas Chalmers called "the expulsive power of a new affection".

Although you may feel you have exhausted all medical avenues, don't forget to think laterally (a very useful skill in general practice). Is there a book that might help, or a DVD to watch? Is there a course the patient can go on? Is there a new skill to learn? Would mindfulness help? What about an exercise programme? Would a fresh approach to medication help? Would it be a good idea to ask a colleague for a second opinion to identify any blind spots? And so on.

2. "And your previous doctor did what?"
I must confess I'm a typical man when it comes to getting my hair cut. I'm not of the 'make an appointment' school, but like to just turn up and wait, although not for very long of course. It's always a slight amusement to me when I'm asked who cut my hair last time, asked in a somewhat disdainful way, until I respond by advising the 'stylist' that it was indeed himself!

We need to be particularly careful when seeing a new patient for the first few times. Remember you need to get to know the patient; tread very carefully before you pontificate. The previous doctor likely had reasons why they prescribed a certain cocktail of drugs that seems odd to us, or for not undertaking an investigation which now seems obviously needed to us.

There is no such thing as a typical 51-year-old woman, any more than there is a typical 65-year-old man. Apart from life opportunities, there will be a myriad of things small and large that define this particular person in front of you.

Certainly, evidence-based medicine (EBM) is hugely valuable, but remember that it is based on populations and not on individuals. As the erudite Michael O'Donnell once said on a course I attended with him, after listening to Professor Sackett, one of the gurus of EBM, "It's all very well to talk of evidence-based medicine but I don't have evidence-based patients!"

3. "You really are talking rubbish"
OK, this is only slightly tongue in cheek, but how often have you thought that when a patient provides an explanation of their ills gleaned from the *Daily Mail*, the internet, or a local alternative practitioner? It may sound OK when written by the script writers on *Doc Martin*, but, although entertaining, he is a very dodgy role model.

Think it you may, but there is probably a better way of moving the consultation forward. Having said that, because I know so many of my patients well, I have been known to lean forward putting my head in my hands in mock desperation, after hearing yet another patient blaming all their ills on candida (usually with the emphasis on the second syllable and rhyming with 'indeed').

Nope, be very careful not to destroy something that may have become very important to the patient. Be gracious and always bear in mind that it is possible to disagree with someone respectfully. So at the very least, hear the patient out, ask them if they want you to comment (rather than just agree with them), and then try to find words that convey the sense that you share the patient's wish to get well but you're not sure that you can agree with the approach recommended. Give your reasons, and be as objective as possible, so don't say, "Ah you saw Madame Blue for allergy tests? Well, she's with the fairies for starters", even if you think she is. Your reply will usually be along the lines of lack of evidence. Remember you are seeking to maintain a relationship with the patient who wants you to at least be open, and be willing to think laterally. Of course, an approach proposed by a patient's adviser that you deem dangerous or manipulative should be exposed as such and the patient dissuaded firmly but carefully. But otherwise remember that the *placebo* is generally speaking one of our greatest friends in medicine.

For reflection

- How well do you cope with patients who have unusual health beliefs?

- Be on the alert with the next new patient you see who is on a cocktail of drugs from a previous doctor. How do you deal with the situation?

- What do you consider that you might *stop* saying to patients?

6

Only the lonely

Today George, a lively 84-year-old, tells me that last year he climbed Kilimanjaro. This he did in memory of his wife who had died and to raise money for a dementia charity.

Still lively, he tells me of a recent walk over some water meadows near Olney and to a bridge over the river. Whilst loitering there he contemplated playing Poohsticks but decided that it's not much fun on your own. Fortunately, just as he was about to give up, a nun passed by. "Do you fancy a game of Poohsticks?", my rather forward patient asks her. "Oh yes, that would be great fun". And so they played.

What on earth are elderly people doing playing Poohsticks?

As George pointed out, "It's no fun playing on your own."

And so I recall the handful of patients I see each week whose fundamental problem is loneliness. With increasing relationship and marital breakdowns, and long years of widowhood, loneliness is a fact of life for many people. There's much evidence to suggest that loneliness is associated with poor health and negative health outcomes. I'm not sure how to legislate against it, but it reminds me that there is yet another question to ask the patient whose non-specific symptoms baffle me. "Would you say that you are lonely?"

I think if asked with sufficient care and the appropriate timing and with a suitable silence after asking, it may open up possibilities of practical help and advice.

* * *

Joy (not her real name) is a single 42-year-old lady who had spent Christmas Day and the next three days entirely on her own. Just one brief phone call to her father on Christmas Day "when he was quite belligerent" was all the human contact she'd had through the season of goodwill.

She was talking to me the other day about her long-standing low-grade depression. When asked how she had been over Christmas her eyes moistened and it took a while for her to tell me. Fortunately, her mood has picked up since then and she is doing her best to socialise in the new year.

* * *

How my priorities have changed as I've got older as a GP. When I started I was mainly concerned with what medical diagnosis I might be missing or what the best antibiotic might be for my patient, and yet the 'softer' subjects of loneliness, poor sleep and lack of exercise now increasingly occupy my thinking when I'm trying to find a helpful way forward for the patient.

A recent very helpful article in the *New York Times*[1] (which is very positive about the UK and the seriousness with which we are taking

---

1   *Researchers Confront an Epidemic of Loneliness*, Katie Hafner, *New York Times*, 5 September 2016, available at bit.do/AGP-6a

the problem of loneliness) points out the detrimental effect on general health that loneliness can have.

> *Researchers have found mounting evidence linking loneliness to physical illness and to functional and cognitive decline. As a predictor of early death, loneliness eclipses obesity. "The profound effects of loneliness on health and independence are a critical public health problem," said Dr. Carla M. Perissinotto, a geriatrician at the University of California, San Francisco. "It is no longer medically or ethically acceptable to ignore older adults who feel lonely and marginalized."*

What to do about loneliness?

- Try to find a sensitive way to ask about it. "Do you often feel isolated?" "Have you recently felt lonely?"

- Help your patient admit that it may be a problem, but that it is not a weakness. It is important that the patient does not feel inadequate or embarrassed to admit it. Although loneliness may partly be self-inflicted, there are often other underlying issues such as dysfunctional families and bereavement.

- Prevention is better than cure. Encourage the patient to welcome people into their home, however humble it may seem to be to them. To my mother's great credit she was inviting various people of all ages round for cups of tea and cake right up until her death at 84 years.

- Encourage friendliness. Sounds trite, but to have friends you have to be friendly. Think about this definition of friendship; "a true friend always lets you in and never lets you down". You do have to 'let people in'.

- Advise cultivating friendships across the age spectrum. I think this is particularly important for those of us who might be vulnerable to loneliness in old age. There are a variety of ways of cultivating this, from joining interest clubs such as photography groups or book clubs, to social gatherings like churches or political parties.

- Suggest contacting support groups that exist to help the lonely such as the Campaign to End Loneliness[2]. There are some fabulous resources here, especially the report for Age UK, *Promising Approaches to Reducing Loneliness and Isolation in Later Life*[3], which makes the following point:

  > … *loneliness is a subjective experience. Loneliness is a negative emotion associated with a perceived gap between the quality and quantity of relationships that we have and those we want.*

  > *In this way loneliness is deeply personal – its causes, consequences and indeed its very existence are impossible to determine without reference to the individual and their own values, needs, wishes and feelings. As such, it is also a complex, and often time-consuming, issue to address. However it is an issue that must be addressed due to the far reaching and devastating impacts that it has on those who experience it on a daily basis.*

- You may be able to make specific suggestions according to your knowledge of local events and societies.

---

2   www.campaigntoendloneliness.org
3   *Promising Approaches to Reducing Loneliness and Isolation in Later Life*, Age UK/Campaign to End Loneliness, Jan 2015, available at bit.do/AGP-6b

For reflection

- Can you recall a time of personal loneliness and how it felt?

- Have you thought about asking patients if loneliness could be a problem? Especially the frequent attender, or those with non-specific symptoms?

- Are you aware of local clubs, organisations, churches, etc. in your area that could help support patients suffering from loneliness?

I second that emotion

"For instance, I know all Mr Wilcox's faults. He's afraid of emotion."
Margaret Schlegel in E. M. Forster's *Howards End*

A little while ago one of our receptionists told me that a patient had gone to the desk and said that the GP had wanted a sample of his emotions. Such malapropisms are relatively common amongst patients, although they are usually of the 'depository' or 'sustificate' variety. Anyway, it would be a very progressive GP who would really ask for a sample of the emotions. But patients certainly do bring their emotions to us and we can either allow them or suppress them. How we cope with patients' emotions will go a long way in enabling us to cope with our own.

Another of our receptionists told me that a particular patient had been very rude to her and indeed after he had left the surgery, she had shed some tears. This was unusual for her and I felt I should support her. So I wrote to the patient, who was in his sixties, and advised him of what I had been told and that I would be grateful if he would apologise to her. Upon receipt of my note he was straight to the surgery to see me. Aggressively he denied that he had behaved rudely or in an intimidating way towards her. As calmly as I could I pointed out to him that he was being aggressive towards me, *at that very moment.* He was astonished. "This is how I speak to everybody", was his riposte.

Now, I suspect there was some exaggeration in that, but clearly, he had little insight into how he came across. We talked it over together and I hope I wasn't patronising. I'm grateful to say that he accepted (to a degree) that the receptionist's perception may have been justified. I realise that the outcome may not always be as satisfactory as this one appeared to be. However, addressing rudeness and supporting our staff is vitally important for team morale (and of course we must ensure it is neither us nor our staff who are rude or aggressive), and we must find ways to deal with such situations.

Afterwards it set me reflecting upon how careful we must be when patients' emotions are firing. My patient was agitated, talking fast and loudly and his tone did come across as several notches above assertive and veering into the aggressive. But he really didn't realise it. What was my role?

- I felt I needed to support the receptionist (after I'd listened carefully to her version of the event).

- I wanted to help the patient 'see himself as others see him'. But this was not easy.

- I needed to be careful not just to win the argument.

- I had to be careful not to be patronising by being so in control of my emotions that I was 'cold'.

Months later I felt it right to bring the incident up with him at an unrelated consultation, and asked how he had felt at the time. "Angry, uncomfortable and embarrassed" was his reply. "But I asked my wife if I came across as aggressive very often; 'of course you do' was her confirmation". As a GP it is so important to enlist the help of the spouse whenever you can…. if they're on your side!

❀ ❀ ❀

He had been on a business trip away from home. But instead of hearing him come through the front door, it was the sound of the doorbell that she heard. And then two police officers standing awkwardly, fumbling somewhat for the right words. "Are you Mrs Repton, the wife of Alan?" Their voices seemed to fade away into the nightmare new world that she found herself in. Mrs Repton was now a widow.

He had been driving to work that morning when a commercial vehicle coming the other way had taken a bend too fast and had hit him head-on. He was killed instantly. I had known him for some years as a patient. He was in his late forties and was a serious, somewhat reserved man. It was later that day that I was sitting in the lounge with his widow and their only daughter who had rushed back from college.

The emotional pain was palpable. Their words were few and their quiet love for each other was evident in the brief moments when their gaze was lifted and coincided. The tears flowed, the sobs were intermittent and the sadness filled the room. I wasn't exempt and tried to be fully present in that moment, not thinking about the surgery I was to do later that day, nor the referral I had left undone. It was just right that I was *there*. Not pontificating, not offering trite words of sympathy, nor trying to be uber-professional in my detachment. I recalled the words of the chaplain of Westminster Hospital from my student days, "Don't just do something, sit there".

And so, I did, and shared a tiny part of their pain. Yes, I said a few things before I left. But they were few. I have seen his widow in the street multiple times since that awful day many years ago. Even now our words are few and the greetings are minimal and yet there remains a connection of shared grief which I regard as a sad privilege.

***

He was convinced that bugs were in the bed and causing his extreme discomfort and itch. He was overwhelmingly fearful that he had an infestation. I had taken a medical history, tried to exclude the recognised causes of persisting pruritus, and hadn't seen much on his skin apart from some evidence of excoriation. I had even treated him for scabies which had made no difference many weeks after the treatment. And now in celebratory mode he produced one of the offending bugs.

I carefully looked at it with my dermatoscope. It was a small piece of fibre, probably from an article of clothing.

I told my patient it wasn't a bug, and despite his protestations, did my best to simply confirm the benign cause of his symptoms. Yes, there may have been real bugs originally (although of course unlikely), and yes, I acknowledged to him that I was doing my best to appreciate how worrying the whole experience had been for him. I even tried some gentle humour – I knew the patient very well – and arranged to follow him up for as long as needed.

His fear and anxiety had been growing over the weeks, I had failed to heal him, and now here I was telling him that it was unnecessary anyway. But it didn't ease his fear and he remained anxious for some weeks afterwards.

I guess unless you have experienced persistent intrusive fear it is perhaps hard to appreciate just how debilitating it is. The close cousin of fear is anxiety and I've come to think that although depression is a truly dreadful illness, it sometimes comes second to severe anxiety in its overwhelming effects.

Yes, there is much that will help anxiety, with CBT and mindfulness being vital tools in a GP's toolbox. But we must never underestimate just how paralysing anxiety can be. We shouldn't play it down, nor try the military approach of 'pull yourself together', however tempting that may be.

It's hard to find that sweet spot of sympathy *and* encouragement to enable the patient to change, but as GPs we have a duty to try to find it. It requires much practice, and I suppose many failures. But it's worth continually working at.

For reflection

• Think of times when it would have been better if you had kept silent, or at least not spoken so soon nor so much. How comfortable are you with silence?

• What is your approach to the angry patient?

• What resources could you point the patient to for self-management of anxiety?

• Could you quickly demonstrate to patients how to perform deep muscle relaxation and diaphragmatic breathing?

8

Seeing the world through the patient's eyes?

TV programmes like *Dragon's Den* and *The Apprentice* have popularised the idea of entrepreneurship and business acumen. However, it was the pioneering reality TV series *Troubleshooter*, which began in 1990 on the BBC, which unpacked the challenge of running a business and reviving poorly performing ones. Sir John Harvey-Jones, the former chairman of ICI, presented the series and became associated with the practice of the boss going on to the shop floor. He was practising the age-old adage of 'standing in someone else's shoes'. One of the central themes from the programme was that the workers on the shop floor often had a very good idea of what needed changing to turn the company around, but the management teams had not put themselves in the shoes of the workers. But when they did attempt the change in perspective, some poorly functioning companies were able to turn their prospects around.

We may think that life as a doctor is difficult at times, but life as a patient certainly isn't easy either. And the journey from being a doctor to being a patient is often a salutary one.

I had to consult with a doctor myself recently. She was excellent. But in what way?

- She expressed unhurried interest (how hard this is in an under-doctored NHS where all GPs have far too many patients!).

- She allowed me to tell my story without impatient and unnecessary interruptions.

- She picked up on my personality and adapted accordingly. I enjoy humour and realise this is sometimes fuelled by nervousness. She went a certain way in responding to my humour, neither ignoring nor going along with it too much. That is to say, I think she got the balance right.

- She was both professional and friendly at the same time.

- I left with a feeling of confidence in her.

At the heart of medicine is still the practice of one person talking to another person. It is about communicating by talking to each other. This is in contrast to the trend of the so-called 'millennials' who apparently value *rapid* service over how that service is delivered. They go for speed rather than the necessary slowing down that human contact requires. The manageress of my local excellent coffee shop tells me that hotels in Japan are experimenting with no staff at all on duty in their hotels, since all check-in is automated and any queries are dealt with by FAQs online (presumably poorly paid workers are still changing the sheets). Increasingly in our culture, freshly prepared meals and coffee brewing is also scorned in favour of the speed of the ready meal and instant coffee. And to cap it all, for us GPs, there is the idea of instant self-diagnosis and treatment on Google. Bah humbug I say, people need people. And good connection between them needs time.

I sometimes have to remind myself that *every* interaction with the patient (i.e. the consultation) is important to them, just as every performance on the stage at the theatre matters to the audience even if it is the actor's second performance of the day – it is likely the first time the vast majority of the audience have seen it. It seems that my sensitive human responsiveness is a necessary part of helping the patients on their journey, whether facing a relatively minor acute illness or something more long term.

❊ ❊ ❊

Andrew Drain, a 33-year-old high-flying cardiothoracic surgeon in training, was diagnosed with acute lymphoblastic leukaemia in September 2007. He died peacefully at home in July 2010. In a wonderfully moving book called *Code Red*[1] are published some talks which he gave during his illness based upon the Old Testament Bible book of Job. Towards the end of the book Drain briefly reflects upon how he might have practised differently as a doctor if he had survived his illness, and in the light of his journey as a terminally ill patient.

He suggested three lessons for busy doctors.

Never forget a patient's dignity

Curtains around a hospital bed are not soundproof. It's very difficult to have confidential conversations with loved ones in an open ward. Leaving urine samples next to a patient's bed may be amusing to good friends, but is a source of embarrassment with less close visitors.

There are so many potential situations when we doctors can forget the essential dignity of each human being. We need to be especially thoughtful when we are consulting accompanied by colleagues who are sitting in with us. For some patients, talking to one person knowing that others are listening in can be unsettling. Of course, we all

---

1   *Code Red*, Andrew Drain, 2010, Christian Medical Fellowship, London

have to learn and patients are given the choice to opt out, but many find that difficult to do. Sensitivity is needed.

And what of the patient with dementia in the care home? It's helpful to see photos of them when they were in their prime, and to know what their work and responsibilities have been through life. In other words, who they are now is an amalgam of who they have been. And so Christopher Reeve, the Superman actor, who became tetraplegic from a riding accident, gave his autobiography the title *Still Me*[2]. Preserving a patient's dignity when they appear to have lost it needs all the thought and skill we can muster.

Patients hang on to every word the doctor says

As a doctor I can't remember how many times I would have told patients casually that we would get a chest X-ray or a scan. For me the day continued as normal. I now realise that for the patient it would be a day waiting and thinking about nothing else but the scan.

I find this to be especially true when talking with patients about a referral, and especially when the diagnosis is uncertain. It is perhaps even more important when debriefing with a family after a bereavement. But also, what about discussing risk? At a pre-operative assessment, the anaesthetist casually said to one of my patients before an elective procedure that there was a 2% mortality risk. Afterwards as the patient chewed it over and told himself that he had a 1 in 50 chance of dying, he felt he needed more time to reflect and in fact subsequently decided to defer the operation.

As we may remember from our school biology days, swallowing is not the same as digestion and absorption. Some information takes time to

---

2   *Still Me*, Christopher Reeve, 1999, Arrow, London

process and it may be days later before a patient realises the meaning of what we said. And that can result in anxiety, in an opposite way to the chuckle of suddenly understanding a joke the following day. All the more reason to be as clear and careful and concise as possible in our spoken words.

Doctors should be careful before dismissing patients' and relatives' concerns

For me this was exemplified when Ruth [Andrew Drain's wife] *shared concerns about me with a member of staff. Ruth had seen me every day for weeks and was concerned that something was wrong and that I was going downhill. In a five-minute conversation Ruth was told to stop being a doctor (she was a doctor actually) and just go home and be a good wife. Within days I was admitted to a different hospital with a serious graft versus host disease. I remember as a houseman my professor telling me to listen to the patient – they are usually right!*

This latter point needs to be ingrained in every GP's thought processes. It is particularly relevant when hearing the concerns of a parent about their child. The parent's hunch that 'little Johnny is just not right' will one day save that child (and you) from disaster. OK, they won't always be right (and nor will you), but a too-quick dismissal of a parent or loved one, who knows how the patient *usually* behaves, is always to be avoided.

———————————— **For reflection** ————————————

- What, if anything, is different in the consultation if our patient is a doctor?

- If you have a tendency to feel hurried in your consultations, try to analyse the reasons. What steps might you take to find a better pace?

The next time you see a patient with dementia, think about this poem called *Names* by Wendy Cope[3]:

She was Eliza for a few weeks
when she was a baby –
Eliza Lily. Soon it changed to Lil.
Later she was Miss Steward in the baker's shop
And then 'my love', 'my darling', Mother.
Widowed at thirty, she went back to work
As Mrs Hand. Her daughter grew up,
Married and gave birth.
Now she was Nanna. 'Everybody
Calls me Nanna,' she would say to visitors.
And so, they did – friends, tradesmen, the doctor.
In the geriatric ward
They used the patients' Christian names.
'Lil,' we said, 'or Nanna,'
But it wasn't in her file
And for those last bewildered weeks
She was Eliza once again.

- Read literature in which patients describe their experience of illness. For depression read *Darkness Visible* by William Styron[4]; for migraine, read *A Brain Wider Than the Sky* by Andrew Levy[5].

3 Included in *Serious Concerns*, Wendy Cope, 2002, Faber and Faber, London. Reproduced here with permission from Faber and Faber Ltd
4 *Darkness Visible: a memoir of madness*, William Styron, 2001, Vintage Classics, London
5 *A Brain Wider Than the Sky: a migraine diary*, Andrew Levy, 2010, Simon and Schuster, New York

9

"Take (extra) care"

It's a familiar sign-off, whether it be text or email, or – wonders never cease – even at the end of a *letter*. You know, one of those things on paper with writing on? The advice? To *take care*. Of course, there are a thousand ways in which a doctor needs to take care. Like most colleagues I am always a little affronted when the local hospital tells me to 'think carefully' before I send a patient in for admission. I know what they mean, but somehow it feels like a criticism that I am not usually thoughtful before admitting a patient to hospital. I guess what the hospital authorities mean is take *extra* care, although strictly speaking isn't the 'extra' superfluous? I recall my mother being told by her doctor she must be extra careful when taking her tablets. What, she wondered, did he mean?

Before I tie myself in knots, let's accept that there is such a thing and that there are some particular aspects to our work where extra thought is needed. Take just three examples.

The letter copied to the patient

There is a growing trend to copy patients in on the correspondence between healthcare professionals. I would suggest that like much else in medicine, it is a mixed blessing. On a number of occasions patients have come to see me clutching a letter which has been copied to them. The contents can cause concern, bafflement and even anger which is not really surprising, given they are often terse missives written in medical jargon.

I recall a lady who had undergone a medical procedure at a noted hospital under a well-known professor. His letter to me made reference to a 'terminal artery'. Although clinically the matter he was discussing was not significant, the sight of the word 'terminal' had completely thrown my patient. She assumed that is wasn't just her artery that was terminal, but that she was too.

More recently a patient received a copy of a letter that had come after her recent outpatient visit. There were so many factual inaccuracies in it that it confirmed to the patient the observed lack of focus that the doctor had displayed during the consultation (apart from his seeming lack of interest, he had apparently answered his mobile phone during the consultation).

So, if you are inclined to copy a patient in on a letter about them that you are writing to a colleague, think about the particular words you use and how the patient might perceive and understand them. Words such as terminal, organic, sequelae and functional are not clear in their meaning to the patient, and may generate unnecessary anxiety.

Giving results

The giving of results is a classic situation and one that needs sensitivity and wisdom. Unless you have undergone tests yourself it's hard to fully appreciate just how anxious some patients become whilst waiting for results. Perhaps even worse is the arrangement of 'if you hear nothing that means everything is all right' – how long should the patient wait before assuming everything is all right? I guess most doctors will recall times when that system has failed and a significant diagnosis has been delayed.

So how best to convey results? I guess much depends upon the particular test undertaken. Typically, a patient will ring up and a receptionist will check the notes and convey what the doctor has said. And that's where the problem starts. Comments like 'borderline' or 'abnormal' may be easy to choose from a picking list, but don't lead to easy conversations when the patient asks, "But what does that mean?".

There's no simple answer and you may need an individualised approach for different results for different patients, which is a challenge working within a stretched NHS where GPs simply care for too many patients.

And then there's the aspect of timing. Timing in sport is crucial, whether it be the explosive lift-off from the athletic blocks almost immediately after the gun has gone off, or the apparently effortless cricket shot that results in four runs, or the careful chase for the ball in football so as not to be offside. Timing is crucial in the practice of medicine too. A worrying result conveyed on a Friday afternoon leaves the patient and loved ones with a weekend to stew and no easy way of having a further discussion with their clinician. There's certainly some value in the old adage, 'good news on a Friday, bad news on a Monday'.

After the miscarriage

The loss of a pregnancy results in the whole gamut of emotions for the affected couple, ranging from devastation to an apparent nonchalance. And even within the couple there may be marked differences in the effect it has on them. It's another case demonstrating the need to personalise the approach to the patient. Don't assume that the 30-year-old with three children already who has a miscarriage at 8 weeks in her fourth pregnancy will be philosophical. And conversely, don't necessarily assume that the 20-year-old primigravida who miscarries at 12 weeks will feel that it is the end of the world. As with all bereavements, we must give patients the space to be themselves.

The longer you spend in practice the more you'll realise that nothing should surprise you. Human beings have an infinite capacity for resilience and a fragility that makes you wonder how civilisation has survived.

And there must be many more situations

- The infertile couple visiting you for the first time. There may be considerable emotion tucked into this situation. The man and woman may be reacting very differently to the situation; be very careful not to 'take sides'.

- When prescribing for the elderly. Do you really need to add to their polypharmacy? Are there any medications that can be stopped? I have seen many patients feel so much better after stopping medication (it's almost worth prescribing so that you can encourage symptom relief after de-prescribing!)

- Any symptom that may seem trivial to you, but is not so perceived by the patient.

- If you have just had a stressful consultation, be especially self-aware in the next few consultations. Don't take it out on the patients who follow.

- Before admitting any patient (especially the elderly) to hospital!

──────────── **For reflection** ────────────

- What situations do *you* need to 'take extra care' in?

- What do you think about the practice of copying letters to patients?

- What is your personal approach about how to convey results?

10

Second opinions

After all those years of training, most of us doctors are a little precious about our professional status. I recall a patient detailing her many and varied symptoms to me after which she simply said, "I want to see someone". I paused and gathered myself and as gently as possible replied that she was seeing someone.... me! But no, she meant she wanted to see someone else! I hadn't even got as far as the first opinion before a second opinion was asked for.

However, it's a time-honoured and often perfectly reasonable request for the patient to ask for a second opinion where a medical opinion has already been offered. It's very important that we allow space for the patient to ask for, and get, a second opinion. We should aim to not take it personally, either if the patient wishes to see another GP colleague, or if the patient asks to see a different specialist from the one whose opinion you had arranged. After all, we all have blind spots and sometimes we may share them with specialist colleagues whose approach is similar to our own, and whose opinion may have been affected by the content of our referral.

There are many reasons why the request may be made.

- A dysfunctional consultation

- A lack of confidence in the opinion given

- Limited treatment options

- A doctor who is unable to make a diagnosis

- A condition and treatment so serious that the patient wishes to be sure of their options

- and so on....

' "There should be no ego involved in getting you the best care", I say explicitly when a patient or a family raises the issue of a second opinion. I am speaking to myself as much as to them'. So writes Jerome Groopman, the Professor of Medicine at Harvard Medical School, in his excellent book, *Second Opinions*[1].

❋ ❋ ❋

It was good to take a walk around Olney with my friend Jon the other day, since he'd never been before and there was much to show him. Having previously lived near the river and the water meadows, I was keen to take him there. So we walked past the Mill House and into the fields to be greeted by one of those Constable vistas. "This would have looked the same to Cowper and Newton over 200 years ago," boasted I. "Did they have wind turbines then too?" came the reply.

Now admittedly you have to look very carefully to see the wind turbines, but they are certainly there. It seems my familiarity with the lovely pastoral scene had obscured what I happily ignored. I couldn't see for looking.

---

1   *Second Opinions: stories of intuition and choice in the changing world of medicine*, Jerome Groopman, 2001, Penguin, London

For the purposes of a medical report, I discovered today that I had seen one patient 36 times in the past 12 months. That's a lot of contact and a lot of time for familiarity to be part of the consultation. It occurs to me that if I am going to see a lot of a patient, it's probably worth asking an equivalent of my friend Jon to take a look every now and then. In other words, get a medical or nursing colleague to take a look. They just might see the wind turbines.

On BBC Radio 4's *Thought for the Day* recently the speaker mentioned a phrase that crops up in Shakespeare's *The Tempest*. Prospero is trying to help Miranda with her memory and says, ' *What seest thou else?*' That is to say, there is more to see than she originally thought she could.

Jon and I continued our walk along the river which I have done many times before, walking to the Rec and then back to the surgery. He noticed how still the water was, how low the level was, how green the grass was. I just walked past it, just enjoying being in dear old Olney by the river.

What seest thou else? It's not a bad question to ask yourself at any and every time and circumstance. There's always more to appreciate in everyone and every part of life. And certainly, with the patient you think you know well.

❋ ❋ ❋

A patient request for a second opinion is usually fair enough, but what we are seeing in hospital outpatients and GP surgeries up and down the country is a sort of system-induced second opinion, and sometimes even a third and fourth. It is the patient who wishes to see the *same* doctor who is out of luck. The doctor has left the department, moved to another practice, only works alternate Tuesdays in months ending in a y, or was 'only' a locum, and so on. It must be so frustrating for the patient – whilst I am wary of familiarity in our consultations, there is so much to be said for *continuity*. A recent research paper by the King's Fund[2] states:

> *'The balance of evidence is that relationship continuity leads to increased satisfaction among patients and staff, reduced costs and better health outcomes, although there are some risks and disadvantages that need to be understood and mitigated......, professional leaders must recognise that relationship continuity can no longer be taken for granted, and that GPs must play a more active role in making it possible.'*

Many patients develop a growing confidence in a particular doctor. And the doctor has an increasing understanding of the context of the patient, which in turn has such an impact upon the possible diagnoses (most notably family, occupational and social history, among others), and also the reaction of the patient to their symptoms and their specific health beliefs. Good old Hippocrates knew a thing or two:

> *It is far more important to know what sort of a patient has a disease than what sort of a disease the patient has.*
> Hippocrates of Cos (c. 460–c. 370 BC)

And providing continuity gives the doctor and patient an ability to follow up differing treatment options, adjusting dosages or changing treatment priorities as needed.

❖ ❖ ❖

---

2   *Continuity of care and the patient experience*, George Freeman and Jane Hughes for the King's Fund, 2010, available at bit.do/AGP-10a

It's all about relationships

I recently read Mark Greene's book, *The Best Idea in the World: how putting relationships first transforms everything*[3]. It's a great read and very pertinent to the idea of continuity. Although the author is making a point about politics it might just as well apply to the practice of medicine.

> *The primary role of politicians is to create conditions in which people can flourish as whole human beings... we have pursued a form of capitalism that is much more concerned with economic growth than it is with social impact.*

> *In our high mobility, high turnover culture most of us have fewer friends than our counterparts 50 years ago, and we are much more likely to live more than half an hour's drive away from relatives. And much less likely to work in the same company for 10 years, never mind our whole lives. Continuity builds trust...*

I realise that it is somewhat countercultural, but I would suggest that there is much to gain from doctors remaining in their specific posts as long as possible. Traditionally GPs would stay in the same practice for their entire working lives. In my own practice this has been the case, although of course this may alter. Another significant and somewhat inevitable trend is the move towards more and more GPs working part-time. There are of course many reasons for this. But we need to find a way to compensate for the consequent loss of continuity and do all we can to preserve as much of it as we can. We'll need to be creative, perhaps through meaningful job shares, where the two sharing doctors meet regularly to discuss their patients and decide upon a unified approach. Or at least to spread out the

---

3   *The Best Idea in the World: how putting relationships first transforms everything*, Mark Greene, 2009, Zondervan, Grand Rapids, MI

part-time work evenly across the week. There are more and more portfolio GPs and whilst this may be a means of preserving broad interests and reducing the perceived or real stress of daily general practice, it may have the counter effect of making practising family medicine much less enjoyable than it was to GPs of a previous generation. They were much less likely to be part-time and although they had to contend with 24-hour responsibility (but none of the hassle of QOF, NICE and revalidation, etc.) they mostly look back upon their careers and the relationship that they had with their patients, with satisfaction. It's the same with hospital consultants; they used to stay in post for many years, much as GPs did, but now they move around. It's all rather unsettling for patients.

For reflection

- How well do you cope with the request for a second opinion?

- If you are working part-time, how can you best facilitate continuity?

- How might you empathise with patients who are frustrated at seeing different doctors?

- What do you and your patients value more, access or continuity?

- How might you approach the patient who is requesting a third and fourth opinion, which is against your better judgement?

11

Silence and small talk

Negative space

One of my more embarrassing moments in life came at the Victoria and Albert Museum in London. For years I have wanted to be able to draw and sketch, and so when I saw an advert for a practical day of drawing for beginners, I happily enrolled along with my equally ambitious son-in-law. We were tutored on shading, perspective and negative space and then were set to work in groups of two around various exhibits at the museum and told to draw what we saw. Yikes!

Having visiting international tourists peering over my shoulder looking at what appeared to be a good imitation of a 6-year-old's drawing was humbling to say the least. I was truly hopeless. But I did learn about 'negative space'.

When seeking to draw a structure we were encouraged not just to look at the lines, but at the spaces between the lines. If trying to draw an arm against the body, instead of drawing the arm we were encouraged to draw the space between the arm and body, and then the space between the arm and the background. This would of course lead to a drawing representation of the arm, but without even realising you'd done it! As the instructor said, "*You need to see the negative spaces in order to draw things in proportion*".

In our consultations, most of us GPs are a little uncomfortable with silences. Consequently we fill the space with questions, comments and explanations which sometimes leave the patient with a sense of not being adequately heard nor understood. As part of our training we might become very skilled in asking questions, and even mastering the art of the open question. But knowing and sensing when to stop the barrage of questions and just to give patients space, or 'negative space', may unlock the consultation door and cement the doctor–patient relationship. How often, I wonder, would a disciplined silence enable the patient to say the very thing that was at the heart of their concerns?

❀ ❀ ❀

'Can't see for looking'

She was 59 years old and had worked for many years in the same local office. She presented with confusion and 'muzzy thoughts'. It was a difficult consultation as I tried to unravel her symptoms. Was it primarily neurological, psychiatric, infectious, malignant, etc.? I felt as though I was getting nowhere. A casual question about her work at a point in the consultation when I was flagging resulted in a delayed response of, "It's OK", and then a sad, dreamy downward gaze. I didn't respond, but merely did my best to look as thoughtful as possible without appearing intense (a sort of Rodin with a touch of Gregory House). Out of the silence, she slowly told me that a few weeks previously she had seen someone in the office stealing a significant amount of money from the petty cash. It was her best friend and she didn't know what to do about it. No wonder she felt confused.

It's often said that a patient will sometimes blurt out the real reason for the visit as they get to the door and say, "By the way, doctor…". I suspect that it doesn't happen that often, and in any event, it wouldn't need to if we mastered those negative spaces and gave permission for our patients to reveal what was really troubling them. They are judging *us*, assessing whether we would understand, and if we would take their concerns seriously.

❊ ❊ ❊

Small talk

Recently I thoroughly enjoyed hearing Alexander McCall Smith talk about his books and his writing. He was relaxed, articulate and in an almost childish way, delightfully funny. Indeed, there aren't many people who laugh at their own stories and yet remain amusing; he effortlessly manages it. But the evening started off by him telling the audience how important small talk is in daily life and in building relationships. He told us that just as baboons spend a lot of time close to each another preening their neighbour, so small talk between people is the vital human equivalent. I confess I haven't contacted David Attenborough to confirm that observation, but it is certainly worth a thought.

Not everyone finds small talk easy. For some it seems such a waste of breath and time, and yet others seem to thrive on it. I would like to make a case for the benefits of small talk even in the time-pressured environment of NHS consultations, where it can seem an irrelevance (although we all know colleagues who would benefit from curtailing their small talk and tangential conversations since it can lead them to run very late!).

Building relationships is at the heart of managing patients in general practice. Although the impression given in the media is of a whole army of patients that just need a one-off consultation for the proverbial cough or similar, the heart and soul of general practice is the caring for patients over a length (and sometimes a very long length) of time. Small talk is going to be an ally in gaining our patients' confidence and possibly even respect. "Do you know what? The doctor often asks how my team is doing…. / how the choir is going…. / how the family are."

Some small talk can seem mechanical and insincere, particularly at the beginning of a consultation, when whilst looking at the screen the doctor asks after the pet dog or how the journey to the surgery was (of course this might be sincere). With experience small talk can be scattered throughout a consultation without losing focus, but generally it is best left until the end, although sometimes the subject of the small talk might be directly relevant to the patient's medical problem.

If small talk isn't your thing, maybe for the patient's sake it's worth at least seeing if you might develop the skill. And what sort of thing is small talk? I would recommend you take a look at an article on the delightfully quirky Art of Manliness website[1] (not just for guys!), from which I adapted the mnemonic **FOR**:

F for Family. Most but not all people love to talk about their family.

O for Occupation. It's the one thing the patient knows about you and that you may not know about them. It may be a source of joy or hassle to them.

R for Relaxation. Ask the patient, 'what do you do to have fun?'

Remember, small talk is not just idle chit-chat with no direct benefit to our consultations. Primarily we are trying to put the patient at ease. We might also find out some key nuggets about their stresses

---

1   Available at bit.do/AGP-11a

and lifestyle at the same time. We could learn that the patient's work is a major cause of stress and anxiety for them, or that they love to exercise in their spare time, or sit on the settee eating doughnuts...

For reflection

- Practise building silence into your consultations. If it feels awkward try to look thoughtful and if necessary say that you just need to give some thought to what has just been said.

- What place does small talk have in your consultations?

- Try using **FOR** if you're struggling with small talk.

12

Shared grief

David had just retired on the dot of his 65th birthday and the next day he presented to me with haemoptysis, weight loss and breathlessness. I'd known him over 25 years although had not seen him often. Most of my contact with his family had been with his wife and her long-standing anxiety, his son, also with anxiety, and his daughter, but mainly through her young children.

He'd worked at the same manual job for over 30 years and was looking forward to 'doing nothing' in his retirement. Sadly that is just how it turned out. He was seen on the two-week wait referral and quickly diagnosed with bronchial malignancy accompanied by a large pleural effusion. Aspiration followed but quickly led to recurrence. Further investigations revealed bony metastases and his deterioration was rapid.

I'm not entirely sure he ever quite grasped the situation or whether he was one of those classic Englishmen who accepted his lot without needing a lot of explanation. Rather like the Tommy of the First World War, he 'just got on with it'.

He died quite quickly at home – I'd scarcely had time to mobilise the palliative care team and district nurses. Wife, son and daughter would gather in the small downstairs lounge whilst David lay uncomplaining upstairs in his bed. With death imminent I gave the family my mobile number and told them it would be OK to call me at any time if he became distressed or, as was more likely, he had died. They were aware of the general arrangements for NHS out of hours care, and appreciated that I couldn't promise them that I would be available, but if possible, I would attend myself, even in the middle of the night.

The following night I received a call from my sister at 2 a.m. to tell me that our mum had been admitted to the acute assessment unit yet again with a fever. She was undergoing chemotherapy for non-Hodgkin lymphoma and over recent months she had begun to lose the battle with her illness. No sooner had I got dressed and gone downstairs than my phone went again. It was David's wife. "I think he's just died". She was calm, matter of fact almost and yet sad. The family knew that my own mother was ill and I told them that I'd just received a call about her, but that I would attend to David first.

As David's wife answered the door she greeted me, "How's your mum?" It was a brief and sweet few seconds as I realised that in that moment, the family cared about me as much as I was trying to care for them. It was a familiar scene. The small family were gathered with other relations drinking tea together. They understood that I wouldn't have time to stay for a drink, but we briefly chatted about how brave David had been. I told them how wonderfully well they had coped with him and cared for him at home. I left and then gradually engaged with my own thoughts and feelings as I drove the ten miles back to see my mother.

Some weeks later David's widow made an appointment to see me. She had been very touched that I had subsequently written to her expressing sympathy and commending their care, but she really wanted to

Changing times

Since the change in the GP contract in 1996 removing 24-hour responsibility, it had been some time since I had visited a patient in the night, other than some night shifts in the early days of the out of hours service. Driving along familiar country roads I reflected on what I had lost since my early days in practice. In my first year, I had attended the local maternity hospital to suture an episiotomy, and for my first ten years I had done all the childhood immunisations. Progressively 999 was used as a first port of call, and ambulances sent to patients who previously would have had a GP attend. I couldn't remember the last time I had injected a patient with intravenous furosemide or intramuscular morphine, waiting and hoping that their acute LVF would improve. Since then patients and their families have become somehow more distant. Care at the time of dying and death has been largely taken over by others and rarely am I called to confirm death. I had become an office worker, albeit very busy and still enjoying the challenge of the practice of medicine, but shared life experiences, friendship and rapport with patients had become harder to establish.

know how my mother was getting on. Mum had indeed picked up a little (although she died some months later). On my way home that evening I called at a village pub for a pint and allowed myself to reflect upon the preceding few weeks. I guess not every GP would want to give out their mobile number and offer to help, nor would they have divulged to the patient's family an illness within their own family. But I had and I didn't regret it.

Since that time, I recall just two other dying patients to whose family I made the same offer and attended in the same way. Truthfully it hasn't been a massive commitment or burden. Patients dying at home are not generally two a penny on the average GP list, and although

I would be circumspect about who and how many such patients to offer myself to, I have been glad of the opportunity and indeed I might say privileged. Some particular experiences build mutual appreciation, and shared care for those dying at home brings back just a little of the sort of rapport that I once knew in my early years of practice. Sharing something of yourself, carefully, selectively and not too frequently humanises us to our patients. It does mean we develop, at least at some level, a kind of friendship with our patients.

It's been said that a friend always lets you in and never lets you down. Our patients are grateful if we never let them down and at times are equally grateful if we let them in.

For reflection

This chapter asks us to consider to what extent satisfaction in our working life relates to physical inconvenience (such as visiting a patient at night, and not getting paid for it!), and allowing patients into our personal and emotional lives. As with other situations in this book, it is not a mandate for how all GPs should behave but merely a challenge to our thinking. What kind of a doctor am I and what kind do I want to be?

- How much of yourself and your circumstances do you reveal to your patients?

- To what extent do you feel it's appropriate to 'let patients in'? Many of us have photos of our families on our consulting room walls. What else might we do?

- How do you feel about giving out your mobile phone number to selected patients at specific times?

- Do you think there is a case for greater involvement by the GP in palliative care and with terminally ill patients?

13

Dying to help

I was brought up by a mother who believed passionately in letter writing. Right up until her death at the age of 84 she was laboriously writing letters every week. And she'd always write one or two drafts before scribing her final copy. Sadly the art of hand writing letters is fading fast, to be replaced by the much less valued email. But as my mum frequently reiterated, people *love* to get letters.

So I was interested to read of an article published recently in the open access medical journal *ecancermedicalscience*[1] which was picked up by much of the print media. It was about the practice of oncologists writing to the bereaved relatives of their patients. As one contributor put it in summary:

> *For doctors, this overlooked practice appears to be an important and now acknowledged part of the cancer story.*

I must say I have for many years tried to remember to write to the recently bereaved and offer my sympathy and words of support; I think it would be a good practice for all GPs. This is another area

---

1   Letters of condolence: assessing attitudes and variability in practice amongst oncologists and palliative care doctors in Yorkshire. *Ecancermedicalscience*, 2016. Available at bit.do/AGP-13a

where longevity in a practice brings its own reward in terms of intimate knowledge of the family relationships and their dynamics. I fully understand that it may be harder for locums and short-stay GPs to get such perspective, but it's worth at least trying.

A few suggestions:

- Don't send a standard letter merely signed by you (or worse, your secretary).

- Do personalise it.

- Try to find something true and interesting about the deceased which you can briefly state. It might be something faintly humorous (although of course humour at such times is incredibly delicate).

- Find a non-trite way of acknowledging the level of pain (for some patients the death of a loved one comes as something of a relief – so no standard, 'you must be devastated').

- Choose your timing. For some as soon as possible after the death would fit, for others two to three weeks later might be more helpful, when the initial attention and busyness has passed.

- Think about hand writing it (currently I dictate but I'm thinking of changing this).

- I prefer headed notepaper to a card. I'm not sure why except that it brings a certain formality into the interaction, along with the warmth of the content.

- It doesn't need to be long.

I know patients appreciate these letters and have had many patients tell me that they read them over and over and keep them for years.

It suggests that our patients *matter* to us and we are not merely professionals with no soul.

❊ ❊ ❊

I visited an old bachelor this week. He was sitting disconsolately on his settee, gently stroking the lifeless body of Charlie, his companion of the last eleven years. The old dog had liver cancer and had passed away during the previous night. He died on the floor of the sitting room. My patient had dialled 999 in the night and the paramedics had come and lifted Charlie up onto the settee; likely one of their more unusual 'emergencies'.

Discussing the situation with the social worker, I was told that "it was only a dog.... you can't really call it bereavement." Oh really?

I'm reminded of some words of C.S. Lewis from *The Four Loves*[2]:

> *To love at all is to be vulnerable. Love anything and your heart will be wrung and possibly broken. If you want to make sure of keeping it intact you must give it to no one, not even an animal. Wrap it carefully round with hobbies and little luxuries; avoid all entanglements. Lock it up safe in the casket or coffin of your selfishness. But in that casket, safe, dark, motionless, airless, it will change. It will not be broken; it will become unbreakable, impenetrable, irredeemable. To love is to be vulnerable.*

❊ ❊ ❊

I recently read *When Breath Becomes Air* by Paul Kalanithi[3]. What a stunning book. A bright, talented young neurosurgeon recounts

---

2   *The Four Loves*, C.S. Lewis, 2012, Collins, London
3   *When Breath Becomes Air*, Paul Kalanithi, 2017, Vintage, London

his journey into medicine and the story of his all too brief career cut short by his cancer and then his grappling with death.

Like Kalanithi, I believe in the power of literature and would love every doctor to read, mark, learn and inwardly digest this book. It's almost a one-sitting read as it's so beautifully written and so thought-provoking. The pilgrimage from dynamic doctor to weak, helpless patient is not easy, but the insights gained would enlighten any practising doctor and especially those who haven't had to grapple with serious illness in their own lives or those of close loved ones.

Patients are our best teachers, and when a doctor becomes a patient they are often given a unique perspective, which can change one's practice for ever. If Henry Marsh (author of *Do No Harm*) thinks every doctor should read this book, I'm not going to disagree. Did I cry? Yep, sitting in Caffè Nero, as the epilogue described his final days and hours, I welled up, thinking of Kalanithi's story, my own mortality and how precious life is. And the reflections by his wife in her early bereavement are a priceless and valuable insight for any GP.

For reflection

- Think about any experience of bereavement you may have had. What means of support did you receive and what was most valuable?

- If you have little or no personal experience of bereavement, consider reading *A Grief Observed* by C. S. Lewis[4], or the Kalanithi book.

---

4   *A Grief Observed*, C.S. Lewis, 2013, Faber and Faber, London

- When you next see a recently bereaved patient, try to arrange a double appointment (or ask if you can bring them back for one) and ask them what has helped them the most. Specifically ask them if they have any comments about the medical care that was given to them and the deceased before, during and after the event.

- Write a letter to the bereaved the next time one of your patients dies.

14

It's all a game of chess

One of the joys of working in general practice at my surgery has been the daily coffee break with my other partners. I nearly always come away having learnt something. Today one of my colleagues suggested that GPs need to be like the knights on a chess board, willing to think laterally and change tack should the need arise. It got me thinking – *the GP as a chess piece*.

The Pawn

Pawns are the basic, unglamorous foot soldiers of the chess game – they can't move far and only work at close quarters. But they are absolutely invaluable to the game.

Much GP work, like any other job, is routine, whether that be reading and writing letters, checking results, or dealing with some (although surprisingly few) straightforward problems. Being a GP can seem unglamorous – I'm sure we've all felt like that sometimes. A hospital consultant once commented to my youngest daughter when she was a surgical foundation doctor, "Oh, so-and-so.... is *only* a GP". Of course, hearing that is rather humbling, even if it was an opinion based upon ignorance!

As a GP it is important that I can identify with patients, and that I know how to travel at their pace, and stay 'close' to them.

Of course, we will not experience everything our patients do, although for me as I've got older it has given me opportunity to experience many of the life events common to our patients, such as bereavement, personal illness, children growing up, and personal dealings with the NHS, 'on the other side', amongst many other things. I know how difficult life can be and am less critical of my patients who are struggling. Staying close to my patients has not only improved my consultations with them, but has made me a better GP all round.

The Castle/Rook

The Castle can move great distances across the board, but only in a straight line. They are powerful pieces, especially when they have a clear line of sight.

I have increasingly made an effort to make contact with colleagues across the country who could advise me on various issues. With the internet and email it's remarkably easy to track down the right person to ask. This in turn has been a great benefit to my patients. Not only can I access expert help, but generally it is immediate and it puts me in a good position to advise my patients accordingly. I recall once reading an excellent book on the management of insomnia by an academic from Harvard, and I was stunned to get a reply to my email query about something he had written, within an hour! I've had the most wonderful and remarkably speedy help from other eminent doctors too. It's a great culture in medicine of mutual support and help, and I hope it will continue.

The Bishop

The Bishop can also cover large areas across the board, but in a diagonal direction only. They can be considered the lateral thinkers of the chess game.

I have found it helpful throughout my career to gain knowledge not just from the obvious – what you might call 'straight in front of me' sources (medical textbooks and lectures, etc.) – but also from novels, popular medical books written for the lay public, and from patients (who may become expert in their particular condition). GPs have a great opportunity to learn about other areas of life from our patients, especially when they have skills from academia, marketing, management, logistics, etc.; what a great resource GPs have, meeting so many different people every day. I think it might have helped me to think laterally in approaching some patients and in turn guide them to find ways forward.

The Knight

Knights have the unique ability to jump over other pieces and, unusually, move at tangents across the board.

As my colleague said, GPs need to be able to be flexible and think around problems. Patients don't always know what their main problem is and we need to talk round and listen well to unpack what they are saying and try to find clarity for them. This may sometimes mean asking a question that initially seems rather angular, but may lead to a particular focus. I think asking great questions is a skill all GPs need to work on. The tangents that some patients seem to take in their responses may actually lead to the nub of the problem, and hence the beginning of an approach to adapt or cope or even relieve whatever ails them.

The Queen

The mighty Queen. She is all-powerful and able to move in all directions, with a full range of skills and abilities.

As GPs, we need to be adaptable to our patients – they really do come in all shapes and sizes and come to us with different backgrounds and circumstances. A 'one size fits all' approach just does not constitute good general practice. Humour helps some patients and alienates others. An investigation is helpful for some but exacerbates anxiety in others. Knowing what to say and do when, and what not to do, is an important skill that must be developed through our careers. The queen has a mighty arsenal; as GPs we have the capacity to build up a toolbox of ideas and approaches such that we might find the closest fit for whatever the patient is looking for help with.

The King

The King is dignified and slow-moving. He shares the Queen's ability to move in all directions, but can only do so one square at a time.

I would suggest that an ability to be suitably serious at times and yet thoughtful always, is necessary. Even making quick decisions about investigations, diagnosis or treatment, can still be conveyed in a considered way. The patient must feel they have been taken seriously, and not just hustled. The rushed patient is seldom the satisfied patient.

Patient-centred medicine is important in its own way, but there are still many times when patients both want, and respond better to, a 'command'. Sometimes patients just want a definitive, kingly, '*just do this*'.

Right, now for the complex characters of mah-jong....

──────────── **For reflection** ────────────

- What do you think are your default styles? Most of us will have a predominant stance that we adopt in our work, although we may have found a way to be adaptable. If you don't know could you perhaps ask your trainer or medical and nursing colleagues (or your non-medical partner)?

- Through your career you may come to realise that even with the same patient, different styles may need to be adopted by you at different times. Maybe sometimes you need to be like the pawn and on another occasion you may need the kingly role. How good are you at adapting and not staying rooted in one mode?

- Is there one 'chess piece' that you could work on over the next few weeks? Try to be self-aware, perhaps even 'score' one of your surgeries in terms of the chess pieces, and notice your default style. Was it always appropriate?

15

The return of vinyl

I'm so glad that vinyl records are making a comeback. Like many of my vintage, I kept all my LPs and it's been great digging them out and playing them again. But surely CDs are better, and Spotify is amazing and so convenient? Yep, I'll agree with that and confess that I'm a keen listener to Spotify. But why vinyl? Let me make a few suggestions.

- The sleeve or covers are just great. They are imaginative, clever and atmospheric. When I see the cover I immediately connect with the content, and even some memories of listening to it previously.

- It's good to have the lyrics within the sleeve – all the best music is enhanced by the words, and the words are given extra power by the music.

- Vinyl just needs more engagement and effort, and is all the better for that. Not always of course, but often enough to make it worthwhile. LPs need to be looked after sympathetically and stored carefully to avoid damage. I have to physically and carefully place the stylus, and I have to get up every 25 minutes or so to change the side of the LP. How short they seem now in the age of streaming.

- Many people comment that there is a clarity to the sound. I'm not sure about that, although with the ear of faith I maybe just get what they are saying.

- After a while vinyl shows its age. There are crackles and pops or even the sound of a fine scratch. Somehow it seems more authentic, if sometimes a little annoying.

Yeah, but what has that got to do with medicine?

Treating patients is never just one-dimensional. It's not just about the consultations or the drugs, or the blood pressure, but it is about the entire interaction between the doctor, the patient and the whole team. In the same way, vinyl is not just about the music, but the sleeve, the lyrics and the engagement that's needed. In other words, it's more *holistic*.

As GPs we need to recognise that the patient has a family, a past, a hoped-for present and future. They have vulnerabilities that the doctor may not have and a context that the doctor needs to know. And all in order to make the doctor–patient interaction more effective on both sides. By considering the patient holistically, there is greater satisfaction for the doctor and perhaps an increased ability to cope with whatever dysfunction the patient is facing.

Vinyl needs looking after. It has to be handled carefully, safely stored away in its sleeve and kept free of dust. And we have to curate our relationships with our patients with a similar amount of care and effort. In the same way, the central act of general practice, the consultation, needs care, attention and thoughtfulness. Such effort will likely be rewarded in more personal fulfilment and greater patient satisfaction.

And what about the crackles? Those scratches that lead to that iconic blip at certain points in that favourite song. Oh yes, they are important. They remind us of the vulnerability and fragility of the human frame. Easily broken, sometimes irreparably so. And also those life experiences that have caused a scar, deeper than the epidermis, that even now produce a recurring 'noise' of sadness, or anger or guilt. It is present in just about every consultation with that particular patient, unspoken perhaps, but always heard by the GP who truly got to know the patient and who has tuned in to it.

But it is also good to be reminded of the vulnerability of the doctor. We are not superhuman. We do make mistakes. We do carry guilt and feelings of what we could have done better, or why we missed that diagnosis. But thankfully, where mutual trust and genuine holistic care exist, our patients are generally so forgiving. We perhaps should join them in forgiving ourselves.

These lines from the famous wedding hymn, 'Praise, My Soul, the King of Heaven', written by Henry Lyte, are a paraphrase of Psalm 103 in which the Psalmist writes, "He knows how we are formed, he remembers that we are dust."

> *Father-like he tends and spares us;*
> *well our feeble frame He knows.*
> *In His hands He gently bears us,*
> *Rescues us from all our foes.*

Over my years of practice I have seen many a patient who is successful in the workplace, and who attends the surgery looking every bit the competent, sorted, and capable professional. And yet as their story unfolds, it becomes apparent that beneath their capable exterior is a human being with frailties like everyone else and who deserves to be treated accordingly. We don't need to be god-like to recognise a feeble frame when we see one. We just need to be open to the possibility.

Doctors and patients. We all have scars. We are all mortal. Thomas Sydenham was a 17th century physician known as the 'English Hippocrates'. He remarked that, "the doctor being himself a mortal man, should be diligent in relieving his suffering patients, inasmuch as he himself must one day be a like sufferer".

The Oath of Maimonides, which some still quote upon qualification, has these words, "may I never see in the patient anything but a fellow creature in pain". As Danielle Ofri comments in her excellent book, *What Doctors Feel*[1], "empathy requires being attuned to the patient's perspective and understanding how the illness is woven into this particular person's life."

The crackles are always there if we listen out for them.

─────────── **For reflection** ───────────

- Practising holistically has become something of a cliché, but how rounded are you in assessing patients?

- Some 'crackles' only become apparent when you have known a patient for a good while. Listen out for them. Perhaps another way of understanding this would be to use the analogy of the bass note, which underlies all that is happening on the surface. For some patients it is good to acknowledge and bring to the surface the bass note from time to time, and perhaps help them move away from it. For others it will take the form of core beliefs (see Lee David's helpful book *Using CBT in General Practice*[2]).

- How has your own experience of illness shaped your practice?

1   *What Doctors Feel: how emotions affect the practice of medicine*, Danielle Ofri, 2014, Beacon Press, Boston
2   *Using CBT in General Practice*, 2nd edition, Lee David, 2013, Scion Publishing, Bloxham

16

The best form of defence?

"We've had a complaint about you."

Perhaps nothing strikes fear more than being greeted with those words by the practice manager. Although some of us may brush them aside, for most of us the anxiety rises as we are handed the letter and read the allegations. More often than not it won't be a serious allegation (which might involve the GMC or even the police), but if it is, the effect upon the doctor, their family and practice can be catastrophic. Even complaints of a lesser order can still stir many emotions and unsettle us; we can begin to doubt our competence and feel paralysed from decision making. Others among us, after receiving what we might perceive as innocuous complaints, react differently and feel simply confirmed in our view that patients are unreasonable and unlikeable.

What is our best defence? For many of us we tinker with the cliché and decide that the best form of defence is defence. That is, we practise medicine in an ever more defensive way, ordering more and more investigations, writing longer and longer notes, spending more time explaining to patients why we are doing what we are doing. There are several reasons why such an approach needs to be challenged.

Say we start to practise excessively defensively and start to order more laboratory tests than we might have done. Medicine throws up a lot of results that are not simply reported as normal, but showing slight deviations from the mean and normal range. This leads on to more uncertainty and confusion for patient and doctor alike. The patient clutching a copy of their results with highlighted results showing a 0.01 figure above the normal range is concerned. "What does it mean?" they may implore, and we usually stutter something like, "Oh, I'm sure it's not significant". Imaging is even more fraught with uncertainties, with the odd opacity noted on chest CT scans, the significance of which is unknown.

So, such defensive medicine may create problems for both you and the patient. But you may argue that you would rather have such problems than miss a diagnosis, and of course missed diagnoses are a major cause of complaint. However, diagnoses are missed either because we didn't do what we would normally do and indeed should have done, in our patient contact (and there may be many reasons for this), or there was a significant gap in our knowledge and experience (for which we may or may not be justifiably culpable).

The best defence

It is of course, hugely important that we remain up to date and constantly review our practice. You should find the time to attend the various update courses and read the helpful literature that the defence organisations produce, but I would like you to consider that perhaps what may prove your best defence throughout your career is the practice of empathy. I would argue that it is not so much specific situations (such as a delayed or missed diagnosis) *per se*, or 'events' as Harold

Macmillan famously said, that lead to complaints, but rather it's how patients or their family *feel* they were treated by their doctor(s). It is rather analogous to the aphorism that employees don't so much resign from their jobs as resign from their managers.

Best treatment

Practising in an empathetic way can have measurable effects upon the patient's health, as Crum and colleagues reported in a recent BMJ analysis, *Making mindset matter*[1]:

> *The qualities of the patient–provider relationship, like empathy and understanding, can also produce measurable physiological improvements beyond the effects of actual treatment by boosting patient expectations, lowering anxiety, increasing psychological support, and improving patient mood. For example, physician empathy has been associated with better clinical outcomes for patients with diabetes, including better haemoglobin A1c and LDL cholesterol control and fewer instances of acute metabolic complications.*

Some years ago, I taught a course in communication skills to third year medical students at a London teaching hospital. It was surprisingly hard work and subsequently gave me some sympathy for all my patients who are teachers who claimed to be exhausted as the end of term drew near. Teaching reluctant learners is draining, and the medical students clearly felt that the time would have been better spent learning about resuscitation skills or how to site a lumbar puncture. During one of the one-to-ones I had with a student who failed to attend much of the course, she told me that her training at Gap clothes store had taught her all she needed to know about

---

1   Making mindset matter. *BMJ*, 2017, 356, available at bit.do/AGP-16a

communication and the only difference was that they expected you to be chirpy all the time.

What I wanted to convey to these students was that when they look back on their career they would realise that the thing that got them through wasn't so much their technical skill and knowledge, hugely important as those are, but rather the ability to relate to patients in an empathetic way. It seems that students still haven't got the message. Writing in the *Student BMJ* in 2015 a second year graduate student mocked the learning of empathy and pleaded, 'we should value competency over empathy'[2]. But such binary thinking is unhelpful. Of course, as doctors we must learn our medicine, but so too must we be students of human behaviour and interactions.

If some critics claim that empathy is ill-defined, "*instead of offering vague courses in empathy training...*"[3], most us know when we have been on the receiving end of an empathetic doctor. Empathy in the context of medical practice encompasses sympathy, and emotional intelligence.

---

2   We should value competency over empathy. *Student BMJ*, 2015; 23. Available at bit.do/AGP-16b

3   ibid.

17

The best form of defence, part 2

Throughout this short book I have alluded to practising in an empathetic way, without necessarily using what I accept is becoming something of a buzzword. But what should we make of empathy?

In the previous chapter I referred to evidence that empathetic doctors may well see measurable improvement in their patients, even in such non-functional conditions as diabetes mellitus. But what is this magical ingredient? Empathy has proved difficult to define, but in his paper published in the journal *Academic Medicine*[1], Professor Hojat from Jefferson Medical College in Philadelphia combines various notions; empathy in a medical context is

> … *a predominantly cognitive (as opposed to affective or emotional) attribute that involves an understanding (as opposed to feeling) of patients' experiences, concerns, and perspectives combined with a capacity to communicate this understanding. An intention to help by preventing and alleviating pain and suffering is an additional feature of empathy in the context of patient care.*

---

1 The devil is in the third year: a longitudinal study of erosion of empathy in medical school. Mohammadreza Hojat *et al.*, *Academic Medicine*, 2009. Available at bit.do/AGP-17a

It seems that some GPs, like the rest of the population, have this more than others, and yet according to Professor Hojat, it's a skill that can be learned. So important is empathy regarded by the American medical insurance industry that 'Empathetics' is now a taught course and medics like Professor Helen Riess from Massachusetts General Hospital are pioneering the way, challenging the assumption that you either have it or you don't. The *Student BMJ* article I mentioned in the previous chapter suggests it just amounts to good manners, but it seems that there is far more to empathy than that.

James Tulsky from Duke University is quoted in a *Washington Post* article by Sandra G. Boodman as saying that "doctors are explaina-holics"[2]. So often our answer to distress is more information, and if a patient just understood their illness better, they would come around. But in reality, bombarding a patient with information does little to alleviate underlying worry.

In her brilliant TED talk[3], Professor Riess draws upon her Empathetics course and teaches the mnemonic **EMPATHY**. Because medical students who have pored over anatomy books like that way of learning, she comes up with her own:

Eye contact is so important

Muscles of facial expressions – learn to recognise emotion

Posture matters – standing over a patient's bedside can be intimidating, so sit down!

Affect – learn to gauge the patient's mood

Tone of voice – learn to recognise what underlying emotion it signifies

---

2   Teaching doctors how to engage more and lecture less. Sandra G. Boodman, *Washington Post*, March 2015. Available at bit.do/AGP-17b

3   *The power of empathy*: Helen Riess at TEDxMiddlebury, 2013. Available at bit.do/AGP-17c

Hear the whole person and understand their context

Your response – allow your emotions to respond.

How might practising more empathetically affect us and our practice?

- It may reduce our prescribing

- It may reduce the likelihood of complaints against us

- It will probably increase our sense of job satisfaction

- Our patients are likely to do better in coping with and even recovering from their ailments

- It may even save you time, as you are more likely to get to the nub of a patient's problem and possibly reduce future attendances.

Just recently I saw Gill, a 40-year-old mother, who stumbled to find the words to express why she had made the appointment. Haltingly she told me that her 11-year-old daughter had been removed from her care and passed over to her ex-husband. She was now only allowed 15 minutes' supervised contact over lunchtimes at school. And with Christmas coming up there would be a 2-week break when she wouldn't see her at all. Prior to this the daughter had just alternate weekends with her father. What had Gill done?

A few weeks ago her daughter had seen her in a distressed state and she explained it was because a very close friend was very poorly in hospital as a result of self-harm. Subsequently, when reprimanding her daughter for being late home, the daughter had said that she was going to harm herself too, "because you're a horrible mummy". The girl had told her father and somehow this conversation found its way to the safeguarding team and all hell was let loose.

Gill was distraught and she couldn't concentrate and nor could she think about anything but her daughter and the injustice of it all. And worst of all, she felt powerless. The tears returned and the room fell silent. So what's to be done? Would medication help? And what sort? Beta blockers for the churning stomach, night sedation for the tearful nights? SSRIs for her low mood and anxiety?

I couldn't pretend for one second to have had the same experience, not least because I am a man, and although I'm a father I have never been denied access to my children, nor been involved with the courts over them, nor have I had personal dealings with the safeguarding team. But I can and indeed did try to put myself in her shoes. Over two consultations she told me the story and of her anguish. We agreed that medication wasn't going to help much, but that the support of friends and others would hopefully see her through. I resisted prescribing.

Before you say anything, am I always so virtuous? Of course not. If I'm not feeling 100%, or am stressed myself, I'm more likely to prescribe in this and other situations. But I don't think that negates my point.

Note we are not just talking about sympathy here, which if offered too abundantly can result in more frequent attendance. I would suggest that empathy is a more professional approach which may well include some 'tough love' in how the help is offered.

For reflection

- How empathetic would you think you are, on a scale of 0–10? Maybe ask close colleagues how they would score you. Is it a skill you might develop?

SECTION II

Looking after number one, *or* Stayin' alive

In this second section of the book I would like to offer some advice on how we look after ourselves for what is a demanding career. There are many books about leadership, and most of them are concerned with how to lead others. However, an essential skill for a lifetime in practice is to be able to lead, and care for, ourselves.

Anyone who has watched an in-flight safety message will know that, in the event of an emergency, you are supposed to put your oxygen mask on before attending to others; you simply cannot help others if you are incapacitated. This section shows you the importance of wearing your metaphorical oxygen mask.

I wish you well.

18

Finding the sweet spot

Working in general practice is a wonderful career, but levels of stress can be high and sustained. We have to find a way to keep going, especially when we are struggling with the demands of work. Our temperaments vary and what some of us need to help us through the stresses and strains of life may be the complete opposite of what others among us might benefit from. To try to find ways of coping and even thriving, however, we will need a good dose of *self-awareness*.

We need to be alert to when our patience is flagging and when decision making is getting harder. We need to identify these and other objective signs that the stress of the job is getting the better of us. These signs will vary with each of us and like the driver's blind spot, may not be recognised by us. So all of us need one or two friends or colleagues with whom we can be exceptionally honest and to whom we have given permission to provide insight to us.

When helping patients understand stress and its effects upon us, I have used this very helpful illustration of the stress see-saw (or fulcrum) which is a very useful tool to show how stress can overload us[1].

---

1   Adapted from *Teach Yourself Managing Stress*, Looker and Gregson, 2003, Hodder, London

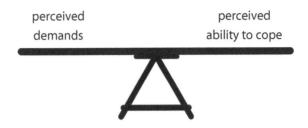

It's all about balancing demands with coping abilities. It is a hugely useful concept for us as practitioners; we should pay close attention to it and apply it to both ourselves and our patients.

We know that a certain amount of stress is good for us and is in fact necessary for how we normally function, but no stress at all causes us to shrivel up. Excess stress (beyond our coping abilities) means we may, sadly, go bust. So we need some stress in our lives, but not too much. We must do all we can to avoid the extremes, and I hope the following chapters will give you some skills and guidance so you can continue to enjoy your job as a GP and not succumb to the stresses it inevitably brings.

I'm all too aware that the previous chapters on patient-facing care can present an ideal that we struggle to live up to much of the time. Yet I'm convinced that enthusiastic, relaxed, chirpy and *balanced* doctors will find patient care much more rewarding than those of us who veer towards over-seriousness and a kind of over-conscientiousness on the one hand, or grumpy resentment on the other. There are, of course, many shades in between. Our patients need us to be the best we can be, but so do our loved ones and friends. You need to accept that there will inevitably be times when the see-saw doesn't balance, but you should at least continue to aim for the sweet spot. So think about how demands may appropriately be reduced, whilst being careful not to leave such a tiny rump of 'what GPs should do', that the job loses its classically holistic nature. And particularly look at ways of increasing your coping abilities.

─────────────── **For reflection** ───────────────

• As you look at the diagram, what is most relevant to you? Reducing demands or increasing your coping abilities?

• Make a decision to work on one aspect over the next month. Write it down on a calendar for a date in one month's time and review how you have done. Be specific. Have you made progress?

19

"I try to look after myself
so I can look after you"

I have found myself saying this a number of times over the years, in differing contexts and to a variety of patients. I contend that it is essential. Looking after yourself has many aspects, of course and, as I wrote in the previous chapter, involves a mix of seeking to increase our coping abilities and reducing the demands. I suspect in the current NHS climate there is a limit to how much we can reduce demands (although there will be areas which can be addressed), so most of what we should work on will be about building our coping abilities.

Knowing your limits is crucial

In the First World War Captain Noel Chavasse was a Royal Army Medical Corps doctor who was the only person to receive the Victoria Cross twice in that conflict. Reading his biography[1] is humbling and unbelievably sad. His dedication to his men was off the scale. Despite the danger, he persisted in his work of rescuing wounded soldiers in no man's land. He continued long beyond the time when he might have legitimately been posted back to the UK to work as

---

1   *Chavasse: double VC*, Ann Clayton, 2006, Pen & Sword Military, Barnsley

a doctor here. He was killed, at the age of 32 years, not long after his engagement to his cousin Gladys Chavasse and just weeks before their intended wedding.

Now, there is no right or wrong about his behaviour, and there were countless other examples of self-sacrifice in that conflict, but there was something about his dedication as a *doctor* that struck me as a warning to us. Maybe others advised him to return home and yet his sense of duty drove him on. After he was killed he could certainly be of no further use to the men of the King's (Liverpool Regiment) whom he loved so much.

You are unlikely to end up tending wounded soldiers in no man's land. However, you should heed the message from this tale. I am sure you want a long, fulfilling and happy career as a GP and you should strive to do your best to achieve this. But please listen to others, and don't be too much of a hero if it's killing you.

For reflection

- Are you too much of a hero? Have you got a messiah complex?

- Do you look after yourself physically? Are you careful about alcohol limits? Are you registered with a GP whom you trust?

20

I'm curious to know if you're curious

One of the challenges of working in general practice, and one that is often not appreciated by our hospital colleagues (especially younger ones) is seeing illnesses at a very early stage. It may be that we are seeing the beginning of a minor self-limiting diagnosis or the foothills of a disease mountain which will overwhelm the patient in a matter of days or weeks. Spotting early warning signs is difficult but it is crucial that we grow in experience of how to do so.

This chapter and the next look at the other types of early warning signs *which we may detect in ourselves*, that may not signify illness, but could be an indicator of problems ahead. We must try to spot these if we are to thrive and survive in general practice.

Lack of curiosity

Lack of curiosity may seem an odd place to start, but it may be a subtle indicator of our career becoming mundane and unfruitful.

Remember our early years at medical school, learning about all sorts of weird and wonderful functions of the human body and what happens when those functions go awry? The amount of material to digest probably seemed overwhelming, but we qualified and began the long journey of learning to be a doctor. My guess is that you don't feel that same enthusiasm for medicine, at least not on a regular basis.

Curiosity about diseases and treatments, and the patients affected by both, naturally waxes and wanes throughout our careers. We experience fatigue, excessive demands, emotional lows and all the gamut of life's experiences. Just about everyone after some years in a job can 'do it with their eyes closed', but medicine deserves eyes wide open as much as we can. Yes, there will be some days when we consciously begin by saying to ourself that we just have to get through the day, and that can be a very reasonable coping strategy on occasions, but if that becomes an established pattern, we need help. Our struggle may not primarily be loss of interest in medicine, but part of a more general malaise. If so, please tell someone; don't withdraw.

How might we rekindle our curiosity?

- Maybe read a medical biography or one of the excellent books written for the general reader on particular diseases and their effects upon history.

- Perhaps find a course on an aspect of medicine that you've always wanted to know more about.

- Arrange to meet with your colleagues (or old chums from medical school) socially and don't be embarrassed to talk medicine sometimes.

- Be around other doctors who still love the variety and challenge of medicine. Ask to sit in on their clinics. I've done this with a number of colleagues (GP or hospital) over the years and they are usually very flattered to be asked. It can really gee you up. Enthusiasm is infectious.

Curiosity will keep us fresh. Try hard not to lose it.

──────────── **For reflection** ────────────

• How is your curiosity quotient?

• What could you do to stimulate it?

• Check out books like

  - *Do No Harm* by Henry Marsh[1]

  - *What Doctors Feel* by Danielle Ofri[2]

  - *The Ghost Disease and Twelve Other Stories of Detective Work in the Medical Field* by Howell and Ford[3]

  - *Toscanini's Fumble* by Harold Klawans[4], a former New York-based neurologist. In fact, Klawans has written several books in the same vein; although they are over 20 years old he tells some wonderful tales of clinical neurology.

1 *Do No Harm: stories of life, death and brain surgery*, Henry Marsh, 2014, Weidenfeld and Nicolson, London
2 *What Doctors Feel: how emotions affect the practice of medicine*, Danielle Ofri, 2014, Beacon Press, Boston
3 *The Ghost Disease and Twelve Other Stories of Detective Work in the Medical Field*, Michael Howell and Peter Ford, 1986, Penguin, London
4 *Toscanini's Fumble and Other Tales of Clinical Neurology*, Harold Klawans, 1990, Headline, London

21

Yes but.....

Another early warning sign of stress getting the better of us is recognising the negative, unhelpful thought patterns that CBT is so helpful in enabling us to identify and challenge. It might be the *all-or-nothing thinking* that may lead us to think that our job is impossible (difficult maybe, but *impossible?*), or other patterns of negative thinking that cloud our judgements and thought processes.

Cognitive behavioural therapy (CBT) is an incredibly useful resource which it is worth all of us getting a real handle on. In the short time we have with our patients in each consultation we can drip feed them the essential concepts. Over a period of time it can really be a wonderfully useful tool in so many ways, whether coping with symptoms of anxiety, depression, obsessions and a whole host of other difficulties which the human frame is susceptible to. As the book title says, the reason *Why Zebras Don't Get Ulcers*[1] is largely because they neither fret over the past nor have anxieties over the future (so far as I know!), and CBT addresses those issues and more.

---

1   *Why Zebras Don't Get Ulcers*, 3rd edition, Robert M. Sapolsky, 2004, Henry Holt, New York

But we need to apply these insights to ourselves. We may be uncomfortable in being compared to a preacher, but St Paul, writing 2000 years ago[2], knew the problem of inconsistency:

> *I run the race then with determination. I am no shadow-boxer,*
> *I really fight! I am my body's sternest master, for fear that when I*
> *have preached to others I should myself be disqualified.*

Catastrophising is another particular pattern of negative thinking that we have to guard against. This is especially a problem when we are inexperienced or have a cautious personality. But it also can become more prevalent when we are feeling overwhelmed by our work. I mentioned in the previous chapter about the importance of being self-aware. Please be aware if you see this change in you.

Catastrophising means we imagine that the worst of possible outcomes will happen, whether it be the blood result we have failed to act upon immediately, or the diagnosis we may have delayed by 24 hours. We need to remind ourselves that the human body is remarkably resilient and the missed blood result will almost certainly not result in the most awful thing imaginable happening. And anyway, if we have worked on our relationships with patients and colleagues, we will likely be forgiven. We are human, and to err is indeed human. Of course, not as a regular occurrence, but at times, yes.

There are many more thinking biases – commonly exploited by fortune tellers and mind readers, amongst others. We all fall prey to them at times. It really is worth learning about this stuff. It'll be enormously helpful for patients and could be a lifesaver for yourself. Check out a book like *Cognitive Behavioural Therapy for Dummies* by Branch and

---

2   1 Corinthians, 9.27, J. B. Philipps translation

Willson[3]. If you can get over being likened to a dummy, you'll find it an excellent, non-demanding read.

———————————— **For reflection** ————————————

- If you tend to catastrophise, how might you learn to challenge your thinking the next time you are aware of it?

- Ask a close friend if you are prone to all-or-nothing (black and white) thinking. How might you modify that tendency?

- Could you try keeping a thought diary of the type recommended in CBT, for a couple of surgeries, to help you gain more insight into your own propensities?

3   *Cognitive Behavioural Therapy for Dummies*, Rhena Branch and Rob Willson, 2010, Wiley, Chichester

22

Get off the bus

Like most patients I'm really not very good at remembering to take medication. And yet you would think that of all people, doctors would be diligent – after all, we know that medication only works if you take it. Amazing, isn't it? Some aspects of medicine are really not rocket science. But what is the problem exactly? Much of it is about *habit* and the difficulties of establishing a new one.

All doctors know the value of reflective practices but few of us engage in them other than fulfilling the mandatory requirements of our training or appraisal. But for self-preservation and personal development, some form of reflection is so helpful. Every now and then it's good to stop, take the pace off life, 'get off the bus' and look back; to reflect on the journey, and try to make sense of it. Please try to get into the habit of adding reflective practice to your toolbox – it will be worth it.

I began diary writing in earnest in 1981 soon after our first daughter was born. Unlike my wife I don't recall small events very well and I wanted to find a way of remembering milestones in our daughters' lives. Not the standard textbook milestones of sitting unaided, walking, etc., but those apparently insignificant moments when one of our daughters first asked me if I'd take her for a picnic, or how much she enjoyed a bike ride, or when our youngest had a general anaesthetic before a dental extraction and seeing her anxious tearful face as she told me she was frightened, and a thousand more memories, thankfully all handwritten in hardback notebooks.

Interspersed with family reflections I found the occasional brief reference to patients. One particular entry, however, was an extended one on a 10-year-old patient who was brought in to see me, weakly groaning and cradled in his father's arms one Monday morning. The lad had become poorly over the weekend and the family, having rung the out of hours service, were given telephone advice. As they entered my consulting room, within milliseconds my neurons fired and I knew I had an extremely ill child on my hands. He was quickly transferred to the local hospital who in turn urgently blue-lighted him to the nearest regional paediatric ITU.

The parents had recently become known to us socially and I felt we should visit the lad to offer support and share in this terrible unfolding. And so, accompanied by my wife I visited the dear young boy, by now ventilated, and with hope for recovery gone. Our distress was dwarfed by the dignified agony of the parents.

That night, back home, I sat and wrote and wrote in my dairy. Pouring out my sadness, trying to express what seemed the futility of it all. I tried to find words for what felt like a horrible failure of modern medicine. I had lots of informal conversations with colleagues in the ensuing weeks, and there were many chats with the heartbroken mum and dad, and I continued being the duty doctor each Monday, always hoping that I would never experience such sadness again. But pouring it all out on the page was, in some unexplained way, a healing balm to me that enabled me to carry on.

——————————— **For reflection** ———————————

- Take one patient encounter this week and write a brief reflection, maybe just 200 words. Record what happened, how you felt, and whether it was something you could have done better or something that worked well that you ought to try again.

- Keep a diary and maybe put a slot in your week of just ten minutes. Block out an appointment, and just write about a patient who made an impression on you. Don't be too analytical or aim for the Booker prize, just write freely and without restraint.

- Use a journal app such as Day One (dayoneapp.com) and set a reminder to write something at a frequency that you think you can manage.

23

Timing is everything

Get to the surgery early so you can start on time. In fact, get there 30 minutes early. I've tried to practise this for many years. That extra 30 minutes catching up, checking results, dictating referrals, etc., can make all the difference to the day. I don't know how many times I have had to remind myself of this. Starting a surgery late is nearly always an effective way of making the ensuing day more stressful.

Avoid procrastination. A number of times I have been asked to do a home visit at about 3 p.m. and have responded by saying that I would go after evening surgery on my way home. It has almost never been a mistake clinically, in that the patient's condition hasn't significantly deteriorated, but it has almost without exception been a mistake emotionally for me. My evening surgery would often have been difficult and by the time I finished I was ready to drop, but I still had the home visit to do. How I regretted my earlier decision.

Try to run to time. Now there are multiple reasons for not running to time (including starting late!) and sometimes it will be completely unavoidable. The challenge is potentially greater in the early years of our career, and the last thing I would want to encourage is speed for the sake of it. We work in an imperfect system (although always remember that the NHS would be a luxury to at least half the world's population), and consulting time can be tight, at 10–15 minutes per patient. It's tough to keep that going through two surgeries in one day, but it's a skill we must develop.

Develop a sense of timing. Use the default time on your computer screen to prompt you. Have a clock behind the patient (careful with your gaze though – most of us can tell if the other person has stopped listening).

If you sense the potential for running over time, *develop language to close the consultation* but without the patient feeling rushed. "Goodness, you have a lot to deal with, I think we need more time to try to help." Or "I really need more time to think through how I'm going to help you. Let's meet again…." If done well, very seldom will the patient feel short-changed.

If a consultation can legitimately be done quickly *don't get side-tracked* on to other things, like gathering data for the computer; your well-being is more important at this point than completing a template. Yet again it's all about balancing your needs with those of your patient. And you'll also have extra time for the patient who needs more than the allotted ten minutes later on.

―――――――――― **For reflection** ――――――――――

- How good are you at running to time? Give some thought to the reasons if this is a problem for you.

- Do you get side-tracked?

- When are you at your best? Morning, afternoon, midweek, etc.? Can you rearrange your surgeries and workload to suit your biological clock?

24

Go off-piste

Medicine is a vast subject and can become all-consuming. In my early years of practice, I was on call for one night each week and for the whole of the weekend, one in three. Looking back that would now be unthinkable to most GPs and yet at the time it felt, and was, normal. But it was satisfying, enjoyable, even if at times wearying. And it was the kind of work one expected. Some thrived and others burnt out through a combination of over-conscientiousness, fatigue and perfectionism.

So much has changed since then, and although the requirement to provide cover for 24 hours a day has gone, the workload has changed. Our days can be intense, long and lacking sufficient breaks. Patient expectations and in consequence complaints, have risen. There is ever closer scrutiny of one's clinical practice, whether that be appraisal, prescribing data or referral rates. And the ubiquitous mobile phone results in a constant state of readiness.

As a doctor you need an outlet, a distraction, and real variety in your life. Think of it as a sort of 'five a day', providing balance and nourishment to your life. You might enjoy sports, and benefit from the physical exercise and the camaraderie that some sports may bring (I'm biased towards rugby!). Making and keeping good friends who have completely differing occupations is so beneficial. Enquiring about a patient's work is not only potentially clinically useful, but is so fascinating. We get the chance to talk with patients who are chimney sweeps, tube drivers, members of the Royalty Protection Group, space scientists and a thousand more occupations. It brings colour to our consultations and our lives.

For me personally, music has played a huge part in my life. I enjoy playing the piano and play most days. For others, playing a more sociable instrument such as guitar, drums or violin and being in a band or orchestra, has been a real joy. Learning a new practical skill like book binding, cooking or sailing takes one's thoughts away from the pressures of medicine and can rejuvenate.

I happen to love reading but I know from my days as an appraiser that not all doctors like to read in their spare time; 'I read enough at work' has been a fairly common response to my question. But for many the joy of reading a well-written novel or biography is a sanctuary and stimulus at one and the same time. Much to my surprise I recently enjoyed an evening class on the novels of Jane Austen. It really doesn't matter what the subject is so long as you find relaxation and joy in something outside of medicine. You need *ballast*. Which, as the dictionary would have it, is 'something to provide you with stability and substance'!

Of course, for those who are part of a family there will inevitably be the joys, responsibilities and trials of family life. And at different ages and stages it will be harder to carve out time for ourselves, but to survive you must at least try.

I recall asking a patient who was about to retire from a lifetime of working in the insurance industry what interests he was looking forward to spending more time on. None, he said, I'm looking forward to doing nothing. That is truly a recipe for disaster.

Remember, you are aiming for balance. It is not that we want to take our medical lives less seriously, but that to enjoy our career more (especially with all the negative talk in the medical and national press), and to be able to give ourselves to it with enthusiasm, we need to find rejuvenators.

For reflection

- What are your main interests outside medicine?

- If family was your answer, do you have any interest or hobby that you could develop?

- What rejuvenates you? Do you give it enough time?

- Do you have enough variety in your life?

- Do you veer towards workaholism or medical minimalism?

25

Good connections

Some clichés are worth holding on to. Take the expression, 'it's not what you know but who you know'. In our early years of medical training and when preparing for professional exams, it is the ability to retain and understand the significance of a vast amount of information that gets us through. It's *what* we know that counts. But I would contend that for surviving and thriving in a lifetime of practice it's not only what you know, but *who* you know that makes the difference.

It should go without saying that within our practices we have frequent opportunities to meet together, although I know that sadly it is not universal. And I don't just mean the partners or practice team formal meetings, but rather those unstructured more relaxed times when over coffee we share apparently insignificant aspects of our lives interspersed with comments and queries about patients and their ills. So much learning can happen in that setting, as much by osmosis as in any more traditional way.

But contemporary practice life tends to reduce the connectedness that we all need. Our modern surgery buildings may have larger consulting rooms and fancy calling systems, but they are not designed with interaction in mind, or that element of bumping into one another that more open-plan buildings facilitated. We may beaver away in our room all day with little personal contact, other than with the patients we see.

One other significant change in the NHS which has resulted in loss of personal connection with hospital colleagues is the rise of the Choose and Book system. No longer does one write, 'Dear Jeremy, this is the patient we were discussing on the phone the either day….'. Now we complete some pro forma with lots of information tucked within it but little to suggest what type of patient we are referring to. And sadly, the generic, 'Dear colleague', or worse, no personal greeting at all, is now commonplace.

Other factors have worsened the situation. Hospital consultants move around far more than in previous years, as do GPs who take short-term contracts as salaried GPs, or work for prolonged spells as locums. And even partners now move on if a better package is offered from a neighbouring practice. Building relationships with colleagues is thus much harder.

What's to be done?

May I suggest that throughout your career you do your utmost to cultivate a friendly professional relationship with as many hospital colleagues as possible? It has been a source of much pleasure and satisfaction to me throughout my career, and often has resulted in better care provided for my patients. There are going to be many times when you just don't know what the next step needs to be in patient care, and even after discussing with your GP colleagues, you still need the additional advice of a consultant who is specialist in a certain area of medicine. It can be enormously helpful in thinking through next steps. And, if appropriate, your colleague may help in overcoming the bureaucracy that can paralyse good patient care, by squeezing your patient into their next clinic, or expediting an investigation. Of course, one can refer in the normal way by letter (although as I say it's becoming increasingly depersonalised), but oftentimes a phone call to someone you *know* is so much more preferable and immediate.

Some of the more delightful experiences I have had in more recent years are when emailing a specialist in a certain field for advice. I may have heard them lecture or read an article or book by them and thought they'd be just the right person to ask for some advice. It's so easy to obtain addresses and nine times out of ten I have been very pleasantly surprised by the prompt, friendly and helpful response – and that despite the fact that I am completely unknown to them. In this way, I have built up a bank of wonderfully helpful specialists in just about every field, some of whom I have now known for several years.

Giving time and energy to this area of our working lives can bear fruit both in decreasing demands upon us and by increasing our coping abilities. Throughout our careers our colleagues are going to be an enormous part of reducing demands upon us, since at the very least a problem shared may be a problem halved (apologies to cliché watchers) and sometimes the demand is not only significantly reduced but even removed altogether. On the other hand, gaining skills and knowledge from other colleagues enables us to bring experience obtained to bear, when facing a similar situation in the future.

———————————— **For reflection** ————————————

- Do you have informal coffee break times with your colleagues?

- If others object that they are too busy, how might you respond?

- Do you have a go-to when faced with a query in cardiology or rheumatology or any other specialty when you need advice?

- Why not leave your room from time to time, make a cuppa for yourself and someone else, have a natter with reception or other staff?

26

Tools in the toolbox

I am rubbish at DIY. For any new (and simple) task I have to buy the necessary equipment. Partly because I don't already have it and partly because I don't know where to find it, even if previously purchased. And yet friends whom I call upon always seem to have the right kit, and have it to hand.

To survive and thrive in general practice you need lots of tools. As with DIY, having access to the right tools will make your job so much easier. It is really worth taking your time to build up a set of tools you can use with your patients, and with yourself. Here's a bunch of mine which I've accumulated and keep well oiled.

- Self-help books for those of your patients who read (OK, not everyone's thing, so I always ask, "Are you a reader?"). I would recommend you read them yourself and get to know the content first.

  - for depression: *Feeling Good* by David Burns. An old book now and rather wordy, but excellent on the disorders of thinking that accompany depression. I suggest just reading the first part.

- for anxiety: *Overcoming Anxiety* by Helen Kennerley. A superb easy to read book with lots of practical suggestions, including a good explanation of CBT.

- for stress: *Managing Stress* by Looker and Gregson. My go-to book for over 20 years. Still my favourite, and countless patients have been helped by this.

- for neck pain: *Treat Your Own Neck* by Robin McKenzie. Another excellent book that has stood the test of time

- for back pain: *Treat Your Own Back* by Robin McKenzie. Ditto.

- for insomnia: *Overcoming Insomnia and Sleep Problems* by Colin Espie, and *Say Good Night to Insomnia* by Gregg Jacobs (this latter is American and is well structured around a 6-week programme developed at Harvard Medical School). Both resources are excellent and have significantly helped many patients stop their night sedation and see their sleep quality improve.

- for autism: *A Parents' ABC of the Autism Spectrum* by Stephen Heydt. As GPs we quickly feel out of our depth here. This book is helpful for us as well as the affected family.

- for irritable bowel syndrome: *Irritable Bowel Solutions* by John Hunter. Full of really useful advice.

- for chronic pain: *Mindfulness for Health* by Burch and Penman. For me this book has been a game changer. Read it first yourself for the brilliant explanation of the nature of pain and the value of mindfulness.

- Get to know the basic principles of CBT so that at least you can give hints and tips to patients. You can't commit to several weeks of 30-minute appointments but you can drip feed. There are masses of resources and online learning tools. An excellent book for you to read is *Two Minute Talks to Improve Psychological and Behavioural Health* by John Clabby. Rather like Jamie Oliver's *Jamie's 30 Minute Meals*, the two minutes here has to be taken with a pinch of salt! Another book would be *Using CBT in General Practice* by Lee David – another excellent read, and a bit more realistic for general practice consultations, especially for identifying patients' core beliefs.

- Learn how to identify and teach diaphragmatic breathing and deep muscle relaxation (see the Helen Kennerley book). It's very simple to demonstrate and is something the patient can do immediately they feel tense and anxious.

- Be flexible in your counselling. Some patients need a problem-solving approach, some will be helped by CBT, others may be helped by taking a more detailed 'life history' and identifying core beliefs and behaviours. And it may be that some patients would be helped by a more *coaching* approach, with its emphasis upon building self-awareness. I have only recently appreciated the value of coaching and suspect that many of us GPs ourselves would benefit enormously from its insights and application.

- Sign up for the excellent GP Update material from Red Whale. This can be accessed online; I open it up at the start of each surgery. A fantastic resource. And their *Lead. Manage. Thrive!* course has brilliant material on managing yourself. See www.gp-update.co.uk for more details.

- Have a ready list of specialists whom you can contact online or by phone.

- Learn from patients and if necessary ask if they would be willing to be expert patients for someone else on your list with a similar condition.

- Point patients to excellent websites, such as the general www.patient.co.uk, or the Living Life to the Full website (www.ltttf.com) for a brilliantly simple explanation of CBT. Alternatively you can use YouTube videos or other videos online. Always watch them first and then build up a library, perhaps including ones which explain exercises such as Brandt–Daroff exercises for BPPV, or how to instil nose drops or perform various musculoskeletal exercises.

- The placebo effect and a patient's attitude towards their illness are some of your most powerful allies. Read *Cure: a journey into the science of mind over body* by Jo Marchant, a phenomenally good book on the power of the mind over the body with very helpful insights into the mechanism of the placebo effect. It has been the most helpful book I have read this past year.

- And don't forget to read these books yourself, for your own health and wellbeing.

─────────────── **For reflection** ───────────────

- What is in your toolbox?

- Do you need to add to it?

- If some of these books are unknown to you, pick the one most relevant to you now. Read, mark, learn and inwardly digest. Then claim brownie points with your appraiser.

- Do you recommend books? Check the Reading Well Books on Prescription website, available at bit.do/AGP-26a. Most public libraries will be able to help patients get hold of these.

Toolbox bibliography

Cure: a journey into the science of mind over body, Jo Marchant, 2016, Canongate, Edinburgh.

Feeling Good: the new mood therapy, David D. Burns, 2000, Harper Collins, London.

Irritable Bowel Solutions: the essential guide to irritable bowel syndrome, its causes and treatments, John Hunter, 2007, Vermilion Publishers, London.

Managing Stress, Terry Looker and Olga Gregson, 1997, Teach Yourself Books, London.

Mindfulness for Health: a practical guide to relieving pain, reducing stress and restoring wellbeing, Vidyamala Burch and Danny Penman, 2013, Piatkus, London.

Overcoming Anxiety, 2nd edition, Helen Kennerley, 2014, Robinson, London.

Overcoming Insomnia and Sleep Problems, Colin Espie, 2006, Robinson, London.

A Parents' ABC of the Autism Spectrum, Stephen Heydt, 2007, Jessica Kingsley Publishers, London.

Say Good Night to Insomnia, Gregg D. Jacobs, 1999, Henry Holt & Co, New York.

Treat Your Own Back, Robin McKenzie, 2011, Spinal Publications, Paraparaumu, New Zealand.

Treat Your Own Neck, Robin McKenzie, 2011, Spinal Publications, Paraparaumu, New Zealand.

Two Minute Talks to Improve Psychological and Behavioural Health, John F. Clabby, 2011, Radcliffe Publishing, London.

Using CBT in General Practice, 2nd edition, Lee David, 2013, Scion Publishing Ltd, Bloxham.

Conclusion

Learning to be a GP is a lifelong task. It can certainly seem overwhelming at the beginning and progressively wearying as the years go by. It's a high stakes job but comes with the opportunity for job satisfaction that many of our patients would love to have.

Nothing worthwhile comes easily, and I can't pretend that there haven't been times when I have felt like giving up. But that next patient whose life and family situation you have contributed to, and who is immensely grateful to you (OK, I know this doesn't happen every day!), somehow gives you energy and enthusiasm to keep going. At such times, if we stop to think, we realise what a privilege it is to be a GP. May I suggest that you avoid medical press of the whingeing variety and try not to talk down your job with colleagues.

Long may the sense of privilege continue as increasingly the organisation of the NHS seems to fragment what GPs do and don't do. The trajectory seems to be squeezing out the holistic nature of our work, offloading onto other health professionals various aspects, so that we will be left with a niche which will bring far less engagement with the patient in their entirety and which has traditionally been the bedrock of British general practice.

I hope it won't sound too self-satisfied to say that patients stand to lose someone who is very important throughout their lives, as we stand to lose much job contentment if we allow the fragmentation to continue. Of course, there will be changes and modifications, but just as you can't get the toothpaste back in the tube, some poorly thought through changes may well be irreversible.

In 1974, during my first year at Westminster Medical School, I attended a lecture by Brian Lacey, the Professor of Bacteriology, on 'The Art of Medicine'. It seems an unlikely topic for a pathologist to address students about, but I have kept my faded copy of the old-style duplicated notes that he handed out. It made several points, the first of which were simply:

Be kind – be sympathetic, compassionate and understanding.

Make no moral judgements.

Always hope (i.e. never despair).

Do not transfer your own anxieties: always reassure.

Soften the truth where necessary without being insincere.

It seems quaint reading it now, but it's nonetheless true. In an ever more impersonal, digital age, with scans and procedures and templates, I can think of no better starting point for us to reflect upon our own practice.

Take good care of yourself and take care of others as best you can. You won't regret it.